the**facts**

Head injury

the**facts**

Head injury

AUDREY DAISLEY
RACHEL TAMS
UDO KISCHKA

OXFORD
UNIVERSITY PRESS

OXFORD
UNIVERSITY PRESS

Great Clarendon Street, Oxford OX2 6DP

Oxford University Press is a department of the University of Oxford.
It furthers the University's objective of excellence in research, scholarship,
and education by publishing worldwide in

Oxford New York

Auckland Cape Town Dar es Salaam Hong Kong Karachi
Kuala Lumpur Madrid Melbourne Mexico City Nairobi
New Delhi Shanghai Taipei Toronto

With offices in

Argentina Austria Brazil Chile Czech Republic France Greece
Guatemala Hungary Italy Japan Poland Portugal Singapore
South Korea Switzerland Thailand Turkey Ukraine Vietnam

Oxford is a registered trade mark of Oxford University Press
in the UK and in certain other countries

Published in the United States
by Oxford University Press Inc., New York

© Oxford University Press 2009

British Library Cataloguing in Publication Data
Data available

Library of Congress Cataloging in Publication Data
Data available

Typeset in Plantin
by Cepha Imaging Pvt. Ltd., Bangalore, India
Printed in China
on acid-free paper by
Asia Pacific Offset

ISBN 978–0–19–921822–6 (Pbk.)

1 3 5 7 9 10 8 6 4 2

Contents

Contributors

Judith Allanson

Consultant in Neurorehabilitation, Community Head Injury Service, Jansel Square, Aylesbury, Bucks

Audrey Daisley

Consultant Clinical Neuropsychologist, Oxford Centre for Enablement, Oxford

Aidan Jones

Consultant Clinical Neuropsychologist, Oxford Centre for Enablement, Oxford

Udo Kischka

Consultant in Neurorehabilitation, Oxford Centre for Enablement, Oxford

Liz Ryan

Relationship and Psychosexual Therapist, Oxford Centre for Enablement, Oxford

Lucy Skelton

Highly Specialist Speech and Language Therapist, Oxford Centre for Enablement, Oxford

Rachel Tams

Consultant Clinical Neuropsychologist, Oxford Centre for Enablement, Oxford

Acknowledgements

We would like to thank:

The many people with head injury and their families, who we have all worked with over the years; learning from them has given us a real insight into the different experiences that families may have after head injury and allowed us to write this book.

The contributors to this book for sharing their experience and expertise with us.

The editorial team at Oxford University Press (Oxford)—particularly Pete Stevenson, Nicola Ulyatt, and Emma Marchant for their patience and guidance.

Professor Derick Wade for generously offering us the opportunity to be involved with this book.

Our families—for their support and understanding.

Foreword

Persons involved in the rehabilitation of individuals who have suffered traumatic brain injury (TBI) or head injury (as it is commonly referred to) have long recognized the need to educate family members about the nature of this complicated brain disorder and the predictable physical, cognitive, and behavioral (including personality) changes that are frequently observed. This book by Daisley, Tams, and Kischka provides the most comprehensive review written specifically for families that I have seen to date.

The text was clearly written with a United Kingdom (UK) audience in mind. Several practical suggestions for helping family members find resources to cope with the problems that a brain-injured loved one may present with exist in the UK. What the authors describe as "the facts" concerning head injury, however, can be meaningfully understood and utilized by family members throughout the world.

This book emphasizes three points. First, family members must be knowledgeable about their relative's head injury, and this requires becoming aware of multiple types of information and familiarizing themselves with new terminology. Even for the experienced professional, this at times can be a daunting task, and yet these authors have gone a long way to simplify rather complicated findings and relationships. While their simplification at times misses points that professionals might wish to emphasize, their book is nevertheless extremely readable and helps families understand in much more detail what the world of traumatic brain injury is like. In this regard, the authors have covered all of the major points that need to be included in educating the family and add an often neglected topic, namely the problems associated with sexuality after TBI. Thus, this brief text is highly comprehensive in nature. Appropriately, the authors warn family members who utilize their book to also seek out appropriate trained professional advice when having specific questions over their loved one. No textbook can cover the variety of complexities that will emerge in a given patient.

Second, these authors discuss practical strategies for managing the cognitive, behavioral, and physical difficulties that confront persons with traumatic brain injury at varying levels of severity. This is extremely helpful.

Third, the authors emphasize throughout the book that family members must "take care of themselves." This, of course, is important advice and every clinician would agree with it. How this is actually done, however, is a complicated process, but it gets family members to think practically over the importance of protecting themselves and that they are not "an unlimited resource" that can be there 24 hours, 7 days a week to care for a person with a brain injury. When family members can appropriately get their needs met while helping their loved one who suffered a brain injury get their needs met, the outcome is almost always more positive for both parties.

This text is easy to read and uses methods of teaching that greatly facilitate providing important facts to family members. Commonly asked questions are highlighted in each chapter and certain "facts" versus "myths" are equally identified. The glossary of terminology may be especially helpful for those who can become confused with the variety of terms that medical and non-medical professionals utilize when describing a person with traumatic brain injury. Knowing what those words mean will help them begin to cope with the inevitable changes that will impact their life forever.

George P. Prigatano, Ph.D.

Preface

Coping with a head injury has been described as one of the most serious challenges that a family can face. This is partly because of its dramatic onset—head injuries happen out of the blue, without any warning and usually in traumatic circumstances. In addition, head injuries can lead to a wide range of problems and have long-lasting consequences which are outside the individual's (and their family's) normal experience. Therefore families can be frightened, distressed, and bewildered by what they are observing and experiencing.

Family members often have many questions about the head injury and what their relative is going through, and may feel isolated and unsupported. If you are in this situation, it is important firstly to know that you are not alone—head injury affects approximately one in 300 families at any one time in England and Wales. There are also professionals and services dedicated to helping those affected by head injury.

This book provides you with essential information about head injury in adults and addresses those questions typically asked by families, guiding you through the head injury journey, from the initial stages when the accident first happens, through early and later treatment, and ending with a discussion of the key long-term issues faced by all those living with head injury. While this can be a very difficult journey to take, our experience of working with head-injured people and their families has shown us that there are things that can make it easier.

By following certain strategies you will better understand what your relative is experiencing, and reduce some of the fear and uncertainty that you and other family members may be feeling. This book provides advice on coping with the range of problems experienced (providing you with information on managing these problems directly, as well as coping with their impact on you), and directs you towards the different types of support services and interventions available to family members (including children). The strategies and suggestions we provide are based on extensive research findings, our own clinical experience and, importantly, what we know has worked for other families.

We want you to use this book in whatever way you find most useful, and to guide your discussions with the professionals involved in your relative's care. You do not have to read the chapters of this book in order. Instead, it is designed so that you can dip into any chapter at any time, allowing you to read about those issues that are most pertinent to you at a particular time. Some sections are written specifically for different family members (e.g. children), and details of other resources and sources of support are given at the end of the book.

Audrey Daisley
Rachel Tams
Udo Kischka
May 2008

1

Coping with head injury: introduction and overview

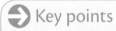 Key points

- According to Headway (the UK's national brain injury association) every year around 1.4 million people in England and Wales will attend A & E as a result of head injury:
  - Each year over a million people attend hospital A and E in the UK following head injury.
  - Around 135,000 of these will be admitted because of the severity of their injury.
  - It is estimated that across the UK there are around 500,000 adults living with long term disabilities as a result of head injury.
- Head injury is one of the most serious challenges a family can face. How families cope with head injury varies enormously. A wide range of coping strategies can be used.
- *Active coping* strategies (such as seeking information and seeking support) are more effective than strategies that involve *avoidance* (e.g. trying not to think about the problems).
- Families require help and support to cope at all stages of their relative's injury, especially in the longer term when they are likely to be the main (or only) source of support to the injured person.

Coping with stressful and traumatic life events is something that almost all families will have to deal with at one time or another. Most of us will experience the death or serious illness of a loved one, the breakdown of a relationship, or the loss of employment, and will need to find ways to cope with the difficult circumstances that arise from these events. Head injury has been described as one of the most serious challenges a family will face, particularly because of its wide-ranging and long-lasting consequences (for both the injured person and their relatives). This book will help to guide you through the 'maze' of head injury so that you feel equipped to cope with the challenges it presents.

What is coping?

In simple terms *coping* refers to the wide range of things that we do or think to try to deal with the situation that we are in. While this might sound straightforward, coping is actually a very complex process. No two people (or two families) are likely to respond to and cope with *even the same situation in exactly the same way.* Furthermore, some coping strategies are more effective or helpful than others, or more appropriate to use at one time than another.

The types of coping strategies that we will use in a stressful situation is partly determined by:

- How we normally cope with stress (i.e. we bring our previous experience to this).
- How others around us cope.
- The amount and type of support we have.
- Factors related to the situation itself (e.g. the nature and severity of your relative's problems).
- The judgements and decisions (sometimes called appraisals) we make about the stressful situation that we are facing. These appraisals are important because they are central to helping us decide what to do next in any given situation (i.e. what course of action, if any, we will need to take):
  - if we judge a situation to be serious and possibly threatening to us we are likely to take one kind of action (i.e. to protect ourselves, or to prevent further harm)
  - if we judge it not to be harmful to us we are likely to take a different course of action (i.e. we may not take any action, or we might just ignore it).

This process of appraisal and trying to work out what an event means for us is likely to take place after head injury and can help us understand why different people (even from the same family) might react emotionally to and cope with similar types of head injury differently.

To complicate matters further, how we cope tends not to be a static process and can change with time, particularly as a situation alters. Therefore, judgements about a situation may alter (again depending on many factors, such as the extent of your relative's recovery or the information you have been given) and your reactions and coping strategies are likely to change alongside this.

Coping with head injury

Considerable research has focused on the vast range of strategies used by families to cope with head injury. The main conclusions are:

- The process of coping with a relative's head injury is constantly changing. Because of the wide-ranging and long-lasting consequences of head injury, families need to draw upon a varied range of strategies to deal with it; some of these strategies might be familiar (as they may have been used previously to manage other stressful situations), while others are new and have to be learned.

- Families often find themselves shifting between different ways of coping depending on the situation facing them, or when a strategy is no longer helpful. Because of this families often say that that it can feel as if they never have a 'grip' on a situation. However, it is also good to try many different ways of coping.

- Adult relatives face the demanding task of helping other family members (particularly children) and friends cope. This can be stressful, especially if they are finding it difficult to cope themselves.

- Families tend to report less distress when they use coping strategies that focus on *active problem-solving* (e.g. actively seeking out information about issues, thinking positively, optimistically, and realistically about a situation, and seeking support, perhaps via counselling).

- Strategies that involve *avoidance* (e.g. trying not to think about the problem, wishing it would go away, or avoiding dealing with the issues associated with it) have been found to be generally less helpful and can lead to higher levels of emotional distress for relatives.

- Families require help and support to cope at all stages of their relative's injury (especially in the longer term when they are likely to be the main (or only) source of support to the injured person). Despite this there is a tendency for services to provide most support in the early and middle stages of recovery but to withdraw in the later stages (at a point when they might be most needed).

What helps in coping with head injury?

There are a number of useful approaches to managing many of the specific head -injury-related problems that your relative might be experiencing. You will find more details about these in later chapters which focus on common post-injury problems. Whatever the type of changes you have noticed in your relative, we know that the following general approaches are often helpful:

1. Become knowledgeable about head injury by seeking information and advice.

2. Know what resources are available, and how to access them.

3. Use strategies to overcome problems. There are many ways in which post-injury problems can be managed, ranging from using simple strategies and aids to altering your environment.

4. Learn to look after yourself and know what forms of emotional and practical support are available to you.

Increasing your knowledge about head injury

You may have heard people say 'knowledge is power', and this is certainly true in the case of coping with head injury. Since most people have no (or little) prior knowledge of head injury, the experience can be confusing as well as distressing. Many relatives have told us that they feel as if they have been transported to an alien planet—they do not know the 'language' of head injury, and so can feel 'stupid' and ill-informed and do not know what questions to ask; thus they worry that they might come across as being uninterested or uninvolved with their relative. Research tells us that seeking information about head injury is one of the most useful coping strategies that families can use. Clear and up-to-date information can help address anxieties, encourage realistic family expectations, and promote more effective coping. Families that are better informed tend to feel more able to cope and often have lower levels of distress. In addition, understanding the nature and extent of your relative's ongoing difficulties can also help you pinpoint particular problem areas and ensure that you are targeting your efforts where they are most needed.

The process of obtaining information after head injury is complex, however, and can be problematic. For example, there tend to be many professionals involved in helping people with head injury and families typically do not know what the different roles of all these people are—again, they do not always know who to seek help from. This can be exhausting, as you might end up having to ask everyone the same question before you find the information you need, or so overwhelming that you ask no one. We try to assist with this throughout this book by trying to explain any technical terms as we use them (but you might also want to refer to the Glossary at the end if you need to find the meaning of something quickly). We have also provided a 'Who's who' section in Chapter 3 to help you navigate your way through the head injury pathway and understand the roles of those you might encounter along the way.

When seeking information, the following can help.

◆ Obtain general information about head injury: this is a good first step in feeling as if you are taking back some control of the situation. There are many excellent websites that can also provide you with general information and facts about head injury. We list these at the end of the book but would like to draw your attention to the **Headway** website at www.headway.org.uk as it is particularly helpful. Headway, the UK's national brain injury association, is a charity set up to provide information and support to people affected by all kinds of brain injury, including head injury. A network of local branches and groups exist throughout the UK offering a wide range of services. There are local variations in what Headway can provide and some of the services we make reference to may not be available in your area. However, Headway have a national helpline number (details provided in back of book). You can use this to gain general information and find out what is available in your area.

◆ Use this general information to help you seek more detailed and personalized information about your relative's head injury and its consequences. Not everyone with a head injury will experience all the problems and issues we go on to describe, and some will experience the same types of problems in different ways and to different extents. Therefore it is helpful to be able to ask very specific questions about your relative's particular patterns of difficulties. With this more detailed information (that is, importantly, tailored to your relative) you will be able to build up a much clearer picture of your relative's strengths and weaknesses, as well as ways to help them. Obtaining this information, being clear about what it means, and remembering it (especially if you are under stress) can be difficult.

If your relative is fully aware of their difficulties (after head injury this may not always be the case), a good starting point is to talk to them and get their perspective on the problems.

Alternatively, talking to the doctor or other health care professionals involved in your relative's care may help you understand what is going on. Make specific time with professionals to have your questions answered, and ask them to write down the key points that have been discussed. Staff members are likely to be busy and you may feel uncomfortable asking for very detailed information; however, doing so will increase the likelihood that you will both understand it and remember it, and so it is likely to be beneficial to you, especially in helping reduce any distress and confusion. It will also save time for staff in the long run.

It is important to take time to absorb the information you have been given and follow up on any issues of concern. It is helpful to write down any questions arising from the initial information you were given, to make time to seek the additional information you require, and to ask for other sources of information (as and when you feel ready to take more on board). The quality, timing, amount, and usefulness of information given to families about head injury varies significantly across services. Therefore it is important to take a proactive approach to seeking the information you need for you and your family, at all stages in your relative's recovery. Be persistent if your questions are not answered adequately.

Become aware of what resources are available

We have already referred above to Headway, the UK's national head injury organization. Your relative's doctor or Headway should be able to provide you with information on the specialist support available locally, such as organizations and support groups that you and your relative can access. You might also be able to access specialist **rehabilitation** services and professionals if they exist in your area. Important contact details are provided at the end of this book.

Use strategies to overcome problems and find ways around your relative's difficulties

As you will read in this book (and as you may already be aware from your own personal experience), many individuals after head injury continue to experience its consequences in everyday life. In the longer term (e.g. once your relative leaves hospital), it is important to find ways around any ongoing problems in order to reduce everyday stress levels within the family. If your relative is accessing support from rehabilitation services, their therapists will be able to advise you on the strategies best suited to your relative's problems. There are also a number of things that you can do to minimize the problems encountered—helping to ensure that your relative is as independent and safe as possible. These general strategies include:

- making simple changes to your home or your relative's work environment (such as labelling drawers, and reducing noise and other distractions)
- drawing on your relative's particular pattern of strengths
- having a clear routine to the day
- using simple aids (e.g. written reminders, alarms, diaries, to-do lists).

These can all help your relative and reduce the stress you may all be feeling.

> Finding ways round ongoing difficulties (sometimes called compensation by rehabilitation professionals) is usually much more effective than searching or working towards a cure or complete recovery.

Some families worry that compensating for the problems (e.g. using a diary to get around memory problems, or using pictures to help your relative communicate) will hinder recovery in some way. We want to reassure you that using aids and making changes to your environment will not hamper your relative's recovery at all.

The many existing resources (leaflets, books, websites) can provide you with practical advice to help deal with the common problems seen after head injury. These will provide a good starting point, but the ideas suggested may need adapting for your relative's specific pattern of difficulties; there is no 'one size fits all' approach. You and your relative will need to try different things out and see what works best for you and your family. In some cases (e.g. if the problems are complex or difficult to understand) you may need more specialist assessment and advice.

Looking after yourself

Head injury is stressful and challenging not only for the individual directly affected but also for other family members. In order to deal effectively with the problems that can arise from your relative's head injury it is important to look after yourself and to know what support is out there for you. This is explored fully in Chapter 9.

2

How the brain works and how it is damaged

➲ Key points

- ◆ Different parts of the brain are specialized in performing certain functions, e.g. moving an arm, speaking, and remembering.

- ◆ Following a head injury, one or more of these functions can be selectively impaired, depending on which parts of the brain are the worst affected.

- ◆ Certain parts of the brain are more vulnerable to damage after a head injury than others and give rise to typical patterns of difficulties.

- ◆ The brain has the ability to recover to some extent after a head injury because undamaged parts of the brain can take over lost functions of the damaged parts. This is called plasticity.

It is much easier to cope with things that we understand. However, the effects of head injuries can be difficult to understand because the brain is such a highly complex organ. As stated in the four principles in Chapter 1, becoming knowledgeable about how the brain works and how it is typically damaged after a head injury is an important first step in understanding your relative's particular difficulties.

The brain
Functions of the brain

The brain is the highest command centre of all the functions of our body:

- ◆ it directs all our actions, such as walking up stairs, typing on a computer keyboard, and talking to a friend

- ◆ it governs our thoughts and feelings

- ◆ it regulates our vital functions (the beating of the heart, breathing, and temperature control) and our hormones.

Different parts of the brain are specialized to perform certain functions: some parts of the brain are in charge of moving an arm, others are responsible for speaking, and others again are active when you remember something. The various parts of the brain have to work together in a highly coordinated way to produce the desired action. For instance, when you talk to someone on the telephone, your ears turn the sounds into electrical signals which are transported to one part of the brain which recognizes them as speech rather than other sounds (such as music or the barking of a dog), and then they are passed on to another part which makes sense of what was said to you. This information is then relayed to yet another part of the brain which forms your answer in your mind, and this activates another area of your brain that controls the muscles you use for forming the words. When you talk to someone face to face, it becomes even more complicated, with all the information from the eyes and the other senses to take in simultaneously. Now imagine driving a car at the same time.

Parts of the brain

The brain weighs about 3 pounds and is an organ of rather soft consistency (a bit like a firm jelly); as such, it is quite a vulnerable structure and can easily be damaged. For protection it is surrounded by the bony skull. Between the brain and the skull are three skin-like membranes and a thin layer called **cerebrospinal fluid** (**CSF**) between these membranes which provide some additional protection to the brain. The CSF is formed within chambers in the brain called ventricles. The brain requires a steady supply of oxygen, glucose, and other substances in the bloodstream to maintain its functioning. The brain has several different parts (Figure 2.1).

The **brainstem** (at the base of the skull) contains the *hypothalamus*, which controls our breathing, heart beat, hormones, and wakefulness. Therefore it is in charge of the body's most vital functions: we can survive damage to the other parts of the brain, but serious damage to the brainstem often leads to coma or death. The brainstem connects the brain to the spinal cord, and it is also involved in moving the muscles of our face and throat.

The **cerebellum** is attached to the back of the brainstem. It plays a role in coordinating our movements, ensuring that the movements of our arms and legs are smooth and precise. It is also involved in keeping our balance while sitting, standing, and walking.

The **cerebrum** is the largest part of the human brain. It has two nearly symmetrical halves called the right and left **hemispheres**. The left hemisphere controls the right side of your body, and the right hemisphere controls the left side of the body. This means that an injury to one side of the brain causes weakness and reduced feeling on the opposite side of the body. In most people, the left hemisphere is responsible for controlling the ability to speak and to understand speech, whereas the right hemisphere helps us to appreciate music

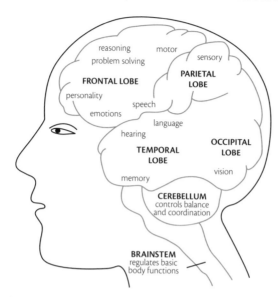

Figure 2.1 The brain

and art. Deep within the hemispheres lie the **basal ganglia** which are involved in performing movements. The surface of the cerebrum is covered by the **cortex**, which has the outward appearance of a series of ridges and troughs. The cortex is involved in intellectual functioning—it is the part of the brain with which we think, remember, and speak. It also controls our sensations and feelings, and the motor cortex controls our voluntary movements. The cortex contains billions of **neurons** or nerve cells, the 'little grey cells' of Hercule Poirot.

The nerve cells or neurons within the brain are connected to other neurons by **axons** (like long fibres) and **dendrites** (like branches of a tree), through which they communicate with each other. They use electrical and chemical impulses to send messages very rapidly from one part of the brain to other parts of the brain and back. The 'grey matter' of the brain refers to the cortex and some parts deep inside the brain containing neurons, and the 'white matter' to those parts that consist of the fibre connections. The neurons also send messages through the spinal cord to other parts of the body. For instance, some neurons activate muscles. Unfortunately, neurons in the brain are quite fragile and can easily be damaged.

The brain and the spinal cord make up our **central nervous system** (**CNS**).

Each hemisphere of the brain has four lobes. Each lobe has its own primary function as well as having to work with other parts of the brain to carry out functions.

The **occipital lobes** are situated at the back of our brain. Everything we see is transformed into electrical impulses in the eyes and transported through the optic nerves and further back to the occipital lobes, which 'make sense' of the incoming information. They turn these electrical impulses into our impression of seeing, for example, the sky, a house, or a person.

The **parietal lobes** are located at the top of the brain. They are involved in a wide range of functions including feeling of touch and pain, carrying out arithmetic, focusing our attention, and orientating ourselves in a building or town (i.e. knowing where we are). They are also responsible for integrating information from different senses, for example when we look at a nice hot cup of coffee which we feel in our hand, smell its aroma, and taste it.

The **temporal lobes** are located at the sides of the brain. The information from our ears is passed on to the temporal lobes, which create our experience of hearing. When we listen to someone talking, the left temporal lobe becomes active and makes sense of what is being said. Furthermore, we use the temporal lobes to store our memories.

The **frontal lobes** are the part of the brain just behind our forehead. They are in charge of our higher-level thinking skills (such as problem-solving and organizing what we do), and initiating and planning our movements and actions. The left frontal lobe is necessary for speaking. The frontal lobes control our emotions and impulses, making sure our behaviour is appropriate to the situation we are in. They also assist us in dealing with new or unexpected situations. The rest of the brain does things pretty much automatically. Imagine, for example, the times that you have driven home from work and when you arrived, you did not remember how you got there. This is because we can do many things, even complex tasks such as driving a car through dense traffic, without really being aware of what we are doing, as if we were on autopilot. Imagine your brain as an aeroplane which gets you from London to New York on autopilot, but during take-off and landing the captain takes over and makes all the decisions. The frontal lobes are like the captain.

Certain parts of the brain work together to produce what we experience as emotions or feelings. These are known as the **limbic system**. Parts of the frontal lobes belong to the limbic system, as does the **amygdala**, a cluster of nerve cells in the temporal lobes. The limbic system will be mentioned later when we talk about the emotional consequences of a head injury.

We are not usually aware of how well the brain works until something goes wrong. When someone has a head injury with damage to the brain, one or more of the brain functions mentioned above can be selectively impaired, depending on which parts of the brain were the worst affected.

What happens in a head injury?

Many people will suffer a head injury at some point in their life, but fortunately in the vast majority it will only be a minor injury. It has been estimated that around one in six people with a head injury requires hospital treatment. In Great Britain, 200–250 people per 100 000 are admitted to hospital with a head injury every year. This means that in a city such as Birmingham with a population of a million, there are 2000–2500 hospital admissions with head injury per year. Young men are much more frequently affected than any other group, although young children and the elderly are also at risk.

Causes of head injury

Road traffic accidents	(about 45 per cent)
Falls	(about 30 per cent)
Accidents at work	(about 10 per cent)
Accidents during recreation/sport	(about 10 per cent)
Assaults	(about 5 per cent)

An injury to the brain can cause a wide variety of symptoms, affecting all areas of our abilities, our experiences, our personality, and our bodily functions. Certain parts of the brain are specialized and are in charge of different functions. If a person has an injury that is limited to just one small part of the brain, he/she may have a very specific problem such as loss of movement in one arm, whereas other functions such as memory and speech can be well preserved (and vice versa). Unfortunately, the very nature of a head injury means that usually the whole brain has been shaken around within the skull. Therefore many parts of the brain are affected to some extent, some more and some less.

How does the brain become damaged in a head injury?

Although the skull and fluid surrounding the brain provide some protection to it during everyday movements, they are insufficient to protect it against large forces. Ironically, the bony skull, despite being there to protect the brain, can add to the damage because it encloses the brain so tightly. When the head is hit from the outside, the brain is thrown around inside the skull with great force. The resulting damage depends on the speed and the direction of the impact, and the location of the injury on the head and in the brain. We will see that some parts of the brain are injured more frequently than others. Additional complications can occur some time after the initial head injury (hours or even days later). These delayed effects can also determine the outcome. A head injury has three phases:

- **First injury**: the initial impact (or damage) which usually occurs within a few seconds.

- **Second injury**: this is determined by the medical condition of the victim in the next few minutes or hours.

- **Third injury**: the consequences of the initial trauma on the person's brain and body over the next days and weeks.

First injury

There are three different types of first injury.

- **Closed head injury**, in which the skull is not penetrated, is the most common head injury. It can happen by acceleration, deceleration, or rotation of the brain within the skull.

  - An **acceleration injury** occurs when the head is at rest and is suddenly thrown back or forwards, for instance when hit by a fist.

  - **Deceleration injuries** typically occur in car crashes, when the head is in motion and suddenly hits an obstacle such as a steering wheel.

  - A **rotation injury** occurs when the head is suddenly turned around very fast.

  Unfortunately, closed head injury does not mean that the injury is not so bad; even closed head injuries can be associated with severe and extensive damage to the brain.

- **Penetrating** (or open) **head injury** occurs when a bullet, a brick, or another object fractures the skull and enters it, and damages the brain directly.

- **Crushing injury** occurs when the head is compressed from two sides, for instance between a car and a wall.

The damage to the brain during the first injury is called **traumatic brain injury** (**TBI**), or sometimes **acquired brain injury** (**ABI**). Damage is usually due to one or more of the following three mechanisms.

- **Contusion** (bruising of the brain): cells of the brain are crushed and destroyed when they are thrown against the inside of the skull. This is usually worst in the brain areas just under the skull at the site where the blow occurred. In addition to the initial contusion at the site of impact, the brain is often also injured at the opposite side as it keeps wobbling back and forth. This is called a **contrecoup injury**.

- **Diffuse axonal injury**: tearing and shearing forces exert their effect throughout the whole brain as it is thrown around inside the skull. The long axons which serve as connections between nerve cells in different parts of the brain are particularly vulnerable to these types of force and they too can be torn and stretched. As this type of damage occurs throughout the brain (and not just in one place), many brain functions can be disrupted to some extent. This is called diffuse axonal injury, and can result in both lasting and temporary brain damage, coma, or death.

◆ **Haematoma** (bleeding caused by rupturing and tearing of blood vessels): bleeding in the brain is quite common after head injury, as arteries running throughout the brain can be ruptured (torn) during this process. This can occur within the brain matter (**intracerebral haematoma**), or between the brain surface and the skull (**subdural haematoma** or **extradural haematoma**). The bleeding exerts pressure on the surrounding parts of the brain, crushing and destroying brain cells in the process.

Second injury

In the minutes and hours after the initial head injury, the medical condition of the injured person may be compromised: the airways may be blocked with blood, so that the brain and the rest of the body do not get enough oxygen. The brain needs a constant supply of blood as this carries oxygen and glucose to the brain cells. If there is blood loss, it can cause a serious drop in blood pressure (*shock*), which also reduces the availability of oxygen and nutrients to the brain. Without oxygen and nutrients, the brain cells cannot function properly and, in time, some of them will die.

Third injury

The head injury triggers processes in and around the brain which can make the situation even worse over the following days and weeks. The most common later problems are **oedema**, **haematoma**, **meningitis/encephalitis**, and **hydrocephalus**. All of these can be life threatening.

Oedema (swelling of the brain)

Most of our body tissue swells when it is damaged, and the brain is no exception. As the brain swells it has nowhere to expand and so it pushes against the skull which can cause further damage. This leads to an increase in the pressure inside the skull (because the space available for expansion of the brain within the skull is limited). The resulting raised pressure (**intracranial pressure (ICP)**) on the brain cells damages them further. The high pressure may also compress arteries in the brain, cutting off some parts of the brain from their blood supply and thus causing **strokes** and even more damage. In severe cases, the pressure can be such that the lower parts of the brain swell and start to push downwards through the only opening in the floor of the skull, thereby compressing the brainstem. This can lead to death.

Haematoma (bleeding)

If a bleed in the brain has occurred but stops, the blood will be reabsorbed by the body's normal cleaning-up mechanisms. However, in some cases the bleeding continues to increase over days and weeks. This happens mostly with bleeds that develop between the brain and skull (subdural or extradural haematomas). The bleeding presses on the surrounding parts of the brain, crushing and destroying brain cells.

Meningitis and encephalitis

◆ Meningitis is an inflammation of the membranes around the brain.

◆ Encephalitis is an inflammation of parts of the brain itself.

These are frequent complications after penetrating injury, whereby bacteria from the outside world gain direct access to the brain. The inflammation destroys brain cells and makes the brain swell. The consequence of the swelling is the same as that described for oedema.

Hydrocephalus

Normally the CSF that is formed within the ventricles of the brain is reabsorbed. Because of the limited space within the skull, this is usually a finely balanced mechanism whereby the amount of CSF produced is identical to the amount that is reabsorbed. After a head injury the mechanism sometimes malfunctions, and the result is increasing pressure within the ventricles, which is called hydrocephalus. The delicate brain cells cannot tolerate the increasing pressure very well and start dying. This situation is not unlike the brain oedema, and it is also life-threatening.

Accompanying injuries

Often the brain is not the only part of the head, or indeed the body, that is affected. Injuries of the eyes and face, hearing loss, broken teeth, and fractures of the skull are common. If the skull has been fractured, CSF can leak out (recognized by fluid running out of the nose or the ear). Other parts of the body can be injured simultaneously with the head injury, such as the spine, arms, and legs, and also the thorax, pelvis, and abdomen including internal organs such as the lungs and kidneys.

There are instances when the injuries to other parts of the body are so severe that the head injury is not noticed initially.

Early clinical symptoms after head injury

Reduced level of consciousness, which is mainly due to widespread damage with diffuse axonal injury throughout the brain, is the most common symptom in the early stages after head injury. The reduction in consciousness can vary greatly: a person with mild reduction of consciousness is awake and talking, but may not know what day it is, a person with more severely reduced consciousness is sleepy and hardly speaks, and a person who remains fully unconscious and unrousable is in a coma.

The level of consciousness is a good indicator of how severe your relative's head injury was. The most widely used method to measure the level of consciousness is the **Glasgow Coma Scale** (**GCS**). It is often used by ambulance personnel and by doctors and nurses in Accident & Emergency (A&E) departments. The injured person is given a score for each of three criteria (Table 2.1).

Somebody who is awake and orientated and talks coherently has a full GCS score of 15, whereas a person who is completely unresponsive is considered as being in deepest coma and has a score of 3. Most people who have had a head injury have some level of reduced consciousness, at least in the early stages. Therefore most have a GCS score somewhere between 3 and 15 immediately after the accident. The reduced consciousness improves quickly if the head injury has been mild, but takes longer to recover with more severe head injury. A person with reduced consciousness requires intensive supervision and treatment in hospital (see Chapter 3).

Table 2.1 The Glasgow Coma Scale

Response	Score
Eye opening	
Opens eyes on his/her own	4
Opens eyes when asked loudly	3
Opens eyes to pain	2
Does not open eyes	1
Verbal response	
Talks normally, fully orientated	5
Confused or disorientated	4
Speaks words but makes no sense	3
Makes sounds, no words	2
Makes no sound	1
Motor response	
Follows instructions	6
Pulls examiner's hand away when hurt	5
Pulls own body part away when hurt	4
Bending of arm when hurt	3
Abnormal extension (straightening) when hurt	2
No motor response to pain	1

In addition to the GCS, there are other ways to estimate the severity of a person's head injury, in particular the length of time the person is unconscious for, and the length of **post-traumatic amnesia** (**PTA**).

In the very early stages of recovery, it is common for individuals to experience PTA, a time of confusion in which they are not fully orientated to their surroundings and what is happening to them, and are unable to take in new information. You may notice during the early days in hospital that your relative finds it difficult to remember everyday events such as family visits. They may not recognize you or other family members and friends, and they might behave in ways that are upsetting to see, for example becoming agitated or aggressive towards others or wandering about the ward. All these behaviours are common at this stage. PTA typically resolves rapidly in the case of mild head injuries (e.g. minutes or hours, rather than days) and your relative should quickly come out of this, becoming more settled in his/her behaviour and more aware of where he/she is. It can last longer in the cases of more moderate to severe head injuries (e.g. days or weeks). For example, if your relative does not remember the accident itself, and the first memory afterwards is the ambulance arriving at the scene, the PTA is probably something like 20–30 minutes. If your relative does not remember anything apart from patchy snippets until he/she was transferred to a rehabilitation centre 3 weeks later, then his/her PTA is 3 weeks. In most cases, this state will improve, but unfortunately, in the case of some severe head injuries, an individual may continue to experience ongoing difficulties and disorientation in everyday life. It can be difficult in such cases to measure the length of time in PTA accurately and to say when this stops (i.e. when the difficulties are judged to be long term and not part of this temporary phase of recovery). The doctors and medical team at the hospital may be able to tell you more about this and give advice on managing these difficulties.

The classification of head injuries into categories of severity is shown in Table 2.2 There is a large range of possible levels of severity of a head injury, and hospital staff tend to use the terms mild, moderate, severe, and very severe when talking about the severity of the injury.

Table 2.2 Severity of head injury according to GCS, length of unconsciousness, and PTA

Severity	GCS score	Length of unconsciousness	PTA
Mild	13–15	Less than 5 min	Less than 1 hr
Moderate	9–12	15 min–6 hrs	1–24 hrs
Severe	3–8	6–48 hrs	2–7 days
Very severe	Not applicable	More than 48 hrs	More than 1 week

Early after the accident, the GCS score gives us a rough estimate of the severity of a head injury. However, the prediction of the final outcome depends partly on how fast the person recovers from the state of reduced consciousness and from the PTA (which are both useful further indicators of the person's chances of making a good recovery). However, we will only know the length of the unconsciousness and the PTA when they are over.

Longer-term symptoms seen after head injury

Once the brain starts to recover, and your relative begins to wake up and become more responsive, it becomes apparent what brain functions he/she has particular problems with, and what he/she can still do well.

The frontal areas of the brain and the temporal lobes are particularly vulnerable in a head injury. This means that the brain functions typically affected after head injury include memory, higher-level thinking skills, such as planning, organization, and problem-solving, and attention. Behaviour and emotional control and expression can also be affected. Because of diffuse axonal injury, thinking speed is often slowed down (as the nerve fibres normally convey information quickly between different areas). In addition to such widespread damage, there can also be additional discrete areas of damage after head injury

Table 2.3 Longer-term difficulties after head injuries

Areas vulnerable to damage	Normal function	Examples of resulting difficulties
Frontal lobes	Problem-solving, initiating and planning activities, controlling aspects of behaviour	Behavioural difficulties Lost initiative/insight Planning problems
Temporal lobes	Hearing, understanding language, memory	Language difficulty Memory problems
Parietal lobes	Feeling of touch and pain, arithmetic, focusing attention, orientating oneself, integrating information from different senses	Attention problems Orientation difficulties
Occipital lobes	Processing what is seen	Visual difficulties
Nerve pathways throughout the brain	Communicating messages rapidly between different brain areas, and between the brain and body	Slower thinking speed Slower reaction times
Brainstem	Breathing, heart beat, wakefulness, moving the muscles of the face and throat	Difficulty swallowing Slurred speech Double vision Reduced consciousness

(e.g. if an artery is torn) and the individual may show specific difficulties on the basis of this, such as loss of speech or weakness of an arm.

Table 2.3 summarizes some of the key difficulties seen, depending on which part of the brain has been damaged. We will discuss these in more detail in Chapters 4–8, together with ways in which they can be managed.

Prognosis: what will the outcome be?

Questions about **prognosis** (i.e. the likelihood and extent of recovery from the head injury) are understandably those most frequently asked by families, and unfortunately are probably the hardest for head injury staff to answer. The severity of the head injury is probably the best determinant of the prognosis, although other factors, such as the location of the injury in the brain, are also important. These will be discussed further in Chapter 3.

Prognosis in mild head injury

The majority (i.e. approximately 85%) of head injuries are classified as mild or moderate, as the initial injury appears minor and they have little or no loss of consciousness. People with a mild head injury usually make a good recovery and can resume 'normal' life within a very short time, often without any resid-ual problems. However, there are a small number of people classed as having a 'mild' head injury who go on to experience significant and often long-lasting problems. This condition is sometimes referred to as **post-concussion syn-drome**, and typically includes:

- headache
- dizziness
- concentration problems
- forgetfulness
- mental and physical fatigue
- irritability.

Recovery from this can be problematic and lengthy, and the person may benefit from advice on rehabilitation. The key message from this is that for some people a 'mild' head injury is not always synonymous with 'mild' problems.

Prognosis in moderate head injury

Approximately 10% of head injuries are classed as moderate, and these patients may require a short hospital stay before being discharged home. Recovery after moderate head injury is usually good, with most people resuming normal life within 6–12 months. However, as with mild injuries, a small number of people with moderate head injuries will experience ongoing problems and may not have resumed all daily activities within a year.

Prognosis after severe head injury

Around 5% of head injuries are referred to as severe or very severe. These patients are likely to require lengthy hospital stays and input from a wide range of professionals. The relatives of people with severe head injury are told to 'expect the worst', even if their relative survives, and have to prepare themselves for long-term problems.

Unfortunately, in a small number of cases after very severe injury the individual remains unresponsive for longer periods of time. They may be unaware of their surroundings or, in some cases, the brain may cease to function completely (a state called brain death). We will begin by looking at these worst-case scenarios.

◆ **Brain death** In a small number of patients, the injuries to the brain are so severe that they are not compatible with life. The swelling of the brain crushes the neurons, and the arteries are unable to transport sufficient blood through the brain. If there is clinical suspicion that the brain has ceased to function, specially trained medical staff perform a series of standardized tests to ensure that there are no reflexes that require brain function. They include widely dilated pupils that do not narrow when a light is shone into the person's eye, and a lack of effort to breathe when the ventilator is disconnected. If there is repeatedly no response on these tests, the patient is declared brain dead. The medical staff may then ask the family for permission to turn off the life-support systems. It is very important to ensure that any questions you have are discussed fully and all concerns are raised. It is appropriate for you to take all the time you need to reach a decision about ending your relative's life support and for you to ask for a second opinion (visit www.waiting.com for further information and advice).

Some patients make only a slight recovery once they come out of coma after severe or very severe head injury, and their state may turn into conditions called vegetative state or minimally responsive state. These states are described below:

◆ **Vegetative state** A small number of patients who have had a particularly severe head injury will remain unresponsive for a longer time. This is called the vegetative state. In this state, the patient has no awareness of what is happening to them or what is going on in the environment around them, but the body still keeps the heart beating and often the breathing going, and a kind of sleep–wake cycle develops. The injured person's basic reflexes continue to function, such as moving a limb to painful stimulation, coughing when a suctioning tube is inserted through the tracheostomy, or even appearing to look around the room. It is understandably difficult for relatives to accept that their loved one who shows these reactions is, in fact, unaware of their presence, particularly, as many of these brain reflexes (such as looking towards someone or reaching out) can appear like meaningful movements.

Because of this, various standardized observations have been produced to try and clarify whether there is any evidence that the head-injured person is aware of their surroundings in any way and to monitor any possible changes in their levels of awareness. These tests need to be carried out by staff who are trained to use them, and so hopefully can provide a much more objective picture of your relative's state at any one time. If it is not possible for these special tests and observations to be carried out by the local team looking after your relative, they may be referred to more specialized rehabilitation professionals for further advice and assessment. If this state persists for more than a month, it is called persistent vegetative state; if it lasts longer than 12 months, it is called permanent vegetative state. The longer-term care of these patients is discussed in Chapter 3.

◆ **Minimally responsive state** People who appear to have some, but little and fleeting, awareness of what is going on around them may be described as being minimally aware or in a low-responsiveness state. They are not in a coma but neither are they fully alert. It is not possible to predict who will improve beyond this state and who will remain minimally aware. Issues relating to communication with people with severe head injury are discussed in Chapter 6.

The states described above are fairly uncommon, and in the majority of cases (even after severe head injury) further recovery is expected.

However, if the patient survives the first few days, it is usually impossible to predict within the first weeks to what extent they will recover. The good news is that even patients with severe head injury often make some progress, particularly if they have access to specialist rehabilitation services.

Further recovery

Fortunately, the brain has some capacity to repair the damage that happened, and undamaged parts of the brain can, in time, take over some of the functions of the damaged parts of the brain. This ability is called brain **plasticity**. In addition, people with head injury and their families can learn new and creative ways of overcoming problems so that the effects of their difficulties are minimized as much as possible.

3

Treatment and recovery after head injury

> ## ⊃ Key points
>
> ◆ Each head injury is different, so each recovery is different.
>
> ◆ There is marked variation in the path that people will follow after their injury, depending on the severity of the injury, the nature of the problems they are dealing with, and the availability of rehabilitation and treatment facilities where they live.
>
> ◆ It is difficult to predict accurately the amount of recovery that will occur after head injury. Factors influencing recovery include severity of the head injury, age, and general health.

Every head injury is different and so each family's experience after the head injury occurs will also be unique. As a result there are many possible outcomes and pathways that an individual (and their family) may take following a head injury (Figure 3.1).

Despite this variation, there are national guidelines in the UK on the type and standards of hospital care that people with head injuries should receive (at the time of writing the most recent of these are the NICE guidelines 2007). In this chapter we outline the most common routes through head injury treatment and recovery, detailing what to expect and the key issues that occur at each stage. However, it is important to acknowledge that as the services available to assess, treat, and support people after head injury in the UK vary enormously, your relative may not be able to access (or need) everything that is described here.

Whatever pathway you follow, it is likely to be the most difficult journey you will ever take with your relative. You may find it bewildering at times, as well as physically and emotionally demanding.

Who's who in head injury treatment and care?

Following your relative's head injury it is almost inevitable that you will be exposed to a startling range and number of professionals who all have a specific

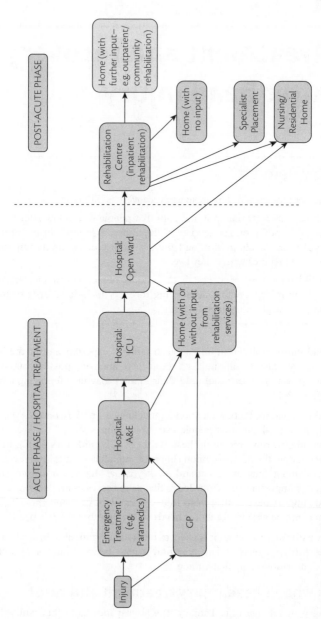

Figure 3.1 Overview of the journey/pathway

role in managing your relative's early treatment and rehabilitation, throughout all stages of recovery. This can be confusing, especially as there often seems to be a lot of overlap and similarities in the work undertaken by professionals. Most professionals work within head injury teams, either in rehabilitation units or in community clinics. They may see you and your relative at home, on a ward, or in clinics. The availability of these therapists and the amount and type of help they can offer will depend on the type of problems your relative has and where you live. The people you might typically encounter are listed in Table 3.1.

Table 3.1 Who's who in head injury care?

Anaesthetists	Specialize in putting patients under anaesthesia, mainly to prepare them for surgery, but sometimes also to calm them down
Clinical neuropsychologists	Psychologists who have trained in health care issues with further specialism in neurological illness and injury. They can assess and treat the cognitive, behavioural, and emotional problems following head injury. They can also provide advice and support to family members. (see www.bps.org.uk)
Consultants in neuro-rehabilitation (doctor)	Specialize in care after the acute stages of illness/injury affecting the brain and/or nervous system. They focus on injured people's needs for ongoing treatment and therapy and often coordinate this work
Counsellors	Specialize in listening and counselling skills. They can offer emotional support at all stages of the recovery process (see www.babcp.org.uk)
Disability employment advisors (DEAs)	Work within the Civil Service and are usually based in job centres. They can offer specialist advice on all issues related to returning to work after illness or injury
Dietician	Experts in the feeding and nutrition of people after illness or injury
General practitioner (GP)	Your usual doctor at your local surgery or health centre. They can refer head-injured people to community- and hospital-based services and may be the key professional involved with people who are not being seen by rehabilitation services
Headway staff	Headway provide a range of day care and support workers throughout the country. They offer long-term support to injured people and their families, often long after professional support ends (visit www.Headway.org.uk)
Neurologists	Specialize in the care of patients with injury or illness of the brain, nervous system, and muscles (such as head injury, stroke, and brain tumour)

Table 3.1 Who's who in head injury care? *(continued)*

Neurosurgeons	Doctors who specialize in surgery involving the brain and nervous system. They use the title Mr or Ms, not Dr
Occupational therapists (OTs)	Health professionals who specialize in helping people with head injury to achieve their maximum level of independence in all aspects of daily life including self-care, work, and leisure activities. They play a key role in assessing and giving advice about specialist equipment (e.g. wheelchair, stair rails) and other adaptations to the home
Orthopaedic surgeons	Doctors who specialize in disease and injury to bones. They can be involved with people who have sustained physical injuries to their limbs or back in their accident. They use the title Mr or Ms, not Dr
Orthoptists	Health professionals who specialize in assessing and treating disorders of the eye and vision. They assess how the eyes work together (binocular vision) and can give advice and aid to manage difficulties that can occur after head injury
Paramedics	Health professionals who are trained to provide acute, sometimes life-saving, help at the site of an accident
Physiotherapists (PTs)	Health professionals trained to help injured people regain and maintain maximum functioning of the body (joints and limbs) through movement and exercise
Psychiatrists	Doctors trained in mental health and emotional issues. Head injury teams may also include neuropsychiatrists (psychiatrists who have particular expertise in problems that occur with neurological illness, such as behavioural problems)
Radiologists	Specialize in performing and interpreting X-rays, CT scans, MRI scans, and similar examination techniques
Rehabilitation nurses	Nurses who are specially trained in the direct care and rehabilitation of people with head injury
Social workers/care managers	Undertake a wide range of activities with injured people and their families and are important when planning discharge home from hospital. They can help arrange carers, access funding, and provide emotional and practical support. Individuals who are pursuing a legal claim against a third party in respect of their injury may have an independent case/care manager appointed; they typically take on a coordinating role, and oversee and monitor the rehabilitation interventions that are taking place. They can sometimes arrange private funding for aids/therapies not readily available via the NHS

Table 3.1 Who's who in head injury care? *(continued)*

Solicitors	Legal experts who may be involved when seeking compensation after injury caused by a third party. Headway can provide a list of personal injury solicitors who deal with head injury
Speech and language therapists (SALTs)	Health professionals who specialize in the assessment and treatment of people with speech and language problems. They aim to help improve speech and language and/or to find alternative ways of communicating after head injury. They are also experts in problems with swallowing
Trauma surgeons	Doctors who are likely to see head-injured people first in A&E units. They are experts in the acute immediate care of injured people and will also arrange for patients to be transferred to the next stage of treatment as appropriate. They use the title Mr or Ms, not Dr

Medical teams are led by consultant doctors (the highest level of qualification). They usually have more junior colleagues working with them with whom you are likely to have more frequent contact. These include specialist registrars (SpRs) (who often have a lot of experience in the field), senior house officers (SHOs) (newly qualified doctors who are undergoing further training, e.g. to become GPs), and medical students. Most teaching hospitals will ask whether you mind students being present during consultations; it is perfectly in order to refuse if you do not want this to happen.

The acute phase
Immediate treatment/getting to hospital

However your relative sustained their head injury, the time immediately afterwards may have been extremely frightening and upsetting for those around the injured individual. If your relative sustained a mild injury (e.g. bumping their head), your first contact with medical professionals may have been through the GP. This may then lead to a hospital admission and contact with other specialist services), or your relative may have been discharged home with no further action.

In cases when injuries are more severe, you may have had to deal with an emergency and life-threatening situation where things happened very quickly. You may not have been sure about what was going on, and you may also have been in a state of emotional shock.

Management at the site of the accident

In many cases, the most important actions immediately after an accident or incident will have been undertaken by bystanders and ambulance crews checking the injured person's **ABC** (airway, breathing, circulation). Ambulance crews will have assessed your relative carefully and noted their level of consciousness at that time using the Glasgow Coma Scale (GCS) (see Chapter 2). Once stabilized, the injured person will have been transferred to hospital.

Management in hospital

Initial assessment in the Accident and Emergency (A&E) department

Once a person arrives at the A&E department, they are examined by doctors and nurses. The following **examinations** are performed.

◆ **Vital signs** Blood pressure, heart beat, breathing sounds of the lung, and temperature are measured. People who suffer a head injury often go into shock with a serious drop in blood pressure, which reduces the availability of oxygen and nutrients to the brain and other parts of the body. Parts of the lungs sometimes collapse, preventing the patient from breathing properly.

◆ **Signs of external or internal injuries** A person who has a head injury often also has other injuries, which can affect virtually every part of the body, including fractures or bleeding inside the abdomen.

◆ **Level of consciousness using the GCS** As discussed in Chapter 2, reduced consciousness is the most common symptom after head injury in the early stages. GCS is the most widely used method to gauge the level of consciousness.

◆ **Reaction of the pupils to light** Normal pupils narrow when a light is shone into the person's eye. If one or both pupils are wide and do not show this reaction, it is a sign of severe injury to the brain with oedema (swelling of the brain).

Further investigations/assessment

If there is any suspicion that the injured person may have suffered fractures, **X-rays** of the head, spine, thorax, pelvis, and/or limbs are taken. If the patient has a moderate or severe head injury, a **CT scan** (computed tomography) is performed. This takes an image of the contents of the skull to show whether there is bruising, bleeding, or swelling of the brain. Other specialist scans, such as **MRI** (**Magnetic Resonance Imaging**), may also be undertaken at this stage.

Ongoing hospital treatment

On the basis of the initial investigations, decisions are made about any further treatment your relative might need.

Management of patients with mild head injury

If the head injury is mild and there are no signs of further injuries, the A&E doctor decides whether the patient should be kept in hospital overnight for observation, or whether he/she can be sent home and told to see the GP within a few days for a follow-up. In most individuals, the initial symptoms and complaints such as headache, dizziness, and sleepiness improve within days or weeks, although sometimes it can take months.

Management of patients with moderate or severe head injury

At this early stage, the emphasis is on stabilizing the person or getting them out of immediate danger. More detailed assessment/investigations (e.g. scans) may be done once this has been achieved. These patients will remain in hospital for further, and more intensive treatments—ranging from surgery to rehabilitation. Such treatments will be focused not only on treating the initial injuries, but also on preventing further complications; they may require intensive and prolonged input from a range of head injury professionals lasting up to many months. The treatment of these patients depends on the findings in the examinations.

- ◆ **Ventilation** Patients who are in a coma are intubated and ventilated. A plastic tube is carefully inserted into their trachea (windpipe) to ensure good access of air into the lungs. If they cannot breathe for themselves, a machine (ventilator) will do it for them by pumping air into their lungs regularly. If a patient needs to be ventilated for a longer period of time, a tracheostomy tube will be inserted through a surgical cut in the front of the neck.

- ◆ **Sedation** Some severely head-injured patients admitted to A&E are confused, restless, and even aggressive (all common in the early stages). They need to be sedated (put to sleep with medication) before they can be intubated. This is also called 'artificial coma'. This is done for the injured person's benefit and protection.

- ◆ **Infusions** Patients are given intravenous (IV) infusions (into the veins) with fluid to prevent them from going into shock, particularly if there was blood loss. Alongside this very basic feeding will also be provided intravenously in the first day or two.

- ◆ Neurosurgeons will be consulted if the **CT scan** shows complications. They decide whether brain surgery has to be performed, which may include drilling a hole in the skull and extracting the haematoma or excess fluid or removing a part of the skull bone in the case of oedema in order to give the swollen brain more space. If the neurosurgeons are concerned that the brain may swell further, they often drill a hole in the skull and insert a small device called an intracranial pressure (ICP) monitor. This is usually removed after a few days.

- ◆ Other injuries sustained in the accident are treated (e.g. fractures are treated surgically, sometimes with metal plates and screws).

This can be a time of great uncertainty and fear for family members, and questions mainly focus on whether or not their relative will survive. Although the procedures described above are essential, they can be upsetting for relatives. You may also be very confused about what the tubes/equipment are for. Once the acute phase is over, ask about the equipment and machinery your relative is attached to and how it is helping him/her. A North American website (www.wait-ing.com), whose primary focus is patients in coma and their families, provides detailed information about intensive care unit (ICU) settings, machinery, and procedures. It is also helpful to familiarize yourself with your relative's medication (ask about side effects and alternatives) and the procedures they are undergoing.

Treatment in the ICU

After acute treatment in A&E, comatose patients are transferred to the ICU where their state is closely supervised by nurses and doctors. Previous treatments are continued, including ventilation, sedation, and infusions. A plastic tube is inserted through the nose into the stomach (nasogastric tube), through which feeding is given.

> ## Treatment in the ICU has several functions
>
> ◆ Monitoring and treatment of head injury-related changes, such as signs of brain oedema or hydrocephalus.
>
> ◆ Continuous monitoring and treatment of changes in basic bodily functions, such as blood pressure, breathing, and blood composition.
>
> ◆ Providing 'round the clock' care.
>
> ◆ Helping the patient to come out of coma. The medical staff on the ICU try to reduce the sedation and, if possible, reduce the ventilation to test whether the patient can breathe unaided.
>
> ◆ Providing appropriate preventative treatments, such as passive movement of the injured person's limbs by physiotherapists to prevent further complications.
>
> The length of stay on the ICU varies greatly from a few days to many weeks.

Epileptic seizures

Some people have epileptic **seizures** or fits within the first few days of their head injury, with individuals who have had penetrating head injury or hae-matoma in the brain being at greatest risk. Seizures occur because the damage in the brain leads to over-excitement of brain cells, which causes them to fire in an uncontrolled fashion. Epileptic seizures are treated with anticonvulsant drugs such as phenytoin; their treatment is discussed in Chapter 4.

Transfer from the ICU to the open ward

Once patients are medically stable they are typically transferred to an open ward. Depending on what is available in your area, this could be a neurology and neurosurgical ward, local stroke unit, trauma and orthopaedic ward, or other general surgery and medical ward. Occasionally hospitals have a dedicated 'head injury' or 'brain injury' ward but this is not the norm. Whatever the name of the ward, the most important thing is that the people looking after your relative are trained to look after individuals with head injury.

Common problems and complications at this stage of recovery

Post-traumatic amnesia (PTA)

As we described in Chapter 2, it is common for individuals in the early stages of recovery to experience a time of confusion. In this condition, patients need very close supervision to ensure that they do not harm themselves or other people. It is important to realize that they are not responsible for their actions. If your relative is aggressive or hostile towards you, he/she is not acting by free will. In dealing with people in such a state, a 'non-confrontational' approach is advisable: it is usually more effective to calm them down or distract them, rather than to try to argue with them or give them orders. In many cases, such patients need to be treated with sedative drugs to calm them down.

Immobility

If your relative remains immobile in bed for weeks, he/she is at increased risk of developing a range of complications:

- pneumonia
- pressure sores of the skin
- contractures of the limb joints (see Chapter 4)
- deep venous thrombosis (DVT) (blood clots in the veins of the legs)
- autonomic function problems (difficulty in controlling body temperature).

Focus of care at this stage

- To continue to manage and monitor head-injury related medical complications.
- To manage and monitor associated injuries such as fractures of the arms or legs.
- To provide assessments and interventions. These early rehabilitation interventions are not likely to be intensive, but rather brief and focused.
    - Physiotherapists start mobilizing patients, helping them first to sit, later to stand and walk.
    - Speech therapists assess whether the patient is safe to swallow food and drink. They also practise speaking if the patient has a problem with this.
    - Occupational therapists retrain patients to dress and wash themselves.
    - Neuropsychologists assess the patients' mental functions, and advise on how to deal with them if they are aggressive.

> ◆ To plan to discharge safely the injured person from acute hospital care—this might involve returning home, seeking alternative care or transferring to another facility for further specialist treatment and rehabilitation.
>
> It is important at this stage that you continue to seek information about the options for further input and care for your relative, getting second opinions if necessary, or begin to think about your relative returning home (if further rehabilitation is not indicated or necessary). Ask questions to help you with the many decisions you will need to make.

The post-acute phase

Leaving the acute hospital

The next stage will depend on how severe the injury was, and what resources are available locally. The most common options are:

◆ transfer to a neuro-rehabilitation centre

◆ transfer to an alternative form of long-term care, such as a nursing home

◆ discharge home:

   ◆ with further input for your relative (this may range from intermittent monitoring to extensive community-based outpatient treatment)

   ◆ without any further input (either because further treatment is not indicated/appropriate or is not available locally).

Although the majority of people with head injury do not receive further care after their injury and are discharged home, rehabilitation is one of the issues most commonly concerning families.

Transfer to a neuro-rehabilitation centre

Neuro-rehabilitation aims to support your relative in their recovery so that they can live as safely and independently as possible. The term simply refers to rehabilitation occurring after neurological illnesses or injuries. This type of support is provided by a team of rehabilitation professionals. The emphasis is on working in collaboration with injured people and their families to achieve meaningful goals that will improve their quality of life. There is a strong focus on seeing the injured person as a 'whole' (not as a set of problems) in their normal everyday context.

Whether occurring in hospital, at home, or in a specialist rehabilitation centre, rehabilitation should be started as soon as possible, and should be provided by a specialist team. Together their goal is to support the patients and their families in:

◆ recovering from their injury

◆ relearning the abilities they have lost, such as moving, speaking, remembering

◆ regaining independence in their everyday life.

To help us understand the impact of an illness or injury on a person, the World Health Organization (WHO) has proposed an International Classification of Functioning, Disability, and Health (ICF) (Table 3.2). This model looks not only at bodily functions, but also at the consequences of the illness or trauma on the person's everyday life, including their ability to care for themselves, as well as the impact on their social roles.

Table 3.2 The WHO Classification of Functioning, Disability, and Health

	Example
Impairment The symptoms and signs, such as weakness of an arm and leg, slurred speech, or forgetfulness	John Miller has a weakness of his right arm
Activity (limitation in activity is also called disability) This looks at activities of daily living (ADL) such as washing, dressing, feeding, continence, and walking	Because of the weakness, he cannot dress and wash himself
Participation (limitation in participation is also called handicap) This refers to changes in the person's social roles within their environment, e.g. their job and their circle of friends	He cannot do his job as a plumber

Although, at first sight, the model may appear rather abstract, it actually has great practical value for the daily clinical work with people after head injury. It shows that even if the impairment (e.g. the weakness of the arm) does not improve sufficiently, your relative may be able to make progress in his/her activities or ability to participate in important social roles. For example, he/she may learn how to dress and wash with the other hand.

Basic principles of therapy used in rehabilitation

- **Practice of an impaired function**: typically this is repetitive, starting with simple tasks and slowly increasing the level of difficulty. For instance, if someone has difficulty moving an arm, they will be encouraged to practice moving this arm. Unfortunately, even with the best will in the world, some people will not regain the use of their arm as it was before.

- Therefore **compensatory techniques** are often used to help the patient to achieve the goal in a different way. For instance, a person with a weakness of the right arm will be taught to dress and wash themselves with their left arm, and a person with memory problems can be encouraged to use memory aids such as a diary.

The different members of the rehabilitation team work together on different aspects of your relative's problems. It is important that they all work together with your relative and yourself towards goals that everyone agrees on. Most neuro-rehabilitation centres encourage family members to become actively involved in the therapies.

During neuro-rehabilitation, the emphasis shifts increasingly towards preparing your relative (and yourself) for returning to live at home. Your relative may be encouraged to spend increasing amounts of time at home. Discharge home from a rehabilitation centre is usually organized in a systematic fashion, and follow-up therapies and care are organized in agreement with you and your relative.

Rehabilitation can be a time of both hope and frustration for your relative and yourself. The process often begins with much optimism (sometimes against advice) for considerable recovery. Sometimes the gains made by injured people following rehabilitation are significant; at other times the progress is modest and slow and families can feel very 'let down' by services. Therefore it is important to be as actively involved in your relative's treatment as possible, so that you are aware of what is realistic and can ask questions about and seek support in dealing with problems.

Rehabilitation can also be a time of conflict within families (e.g. if the family and their relative cannot agree on common goals, or if the injured person is not fully aware of their difficulties) or most commonly with members of the team (e.g. if family members feel that progress is too slow or they do not agree with the team's recommendations). Again, it is helpful to be open about concerns and find ways to work in collaboration with your relative's team.

People may require transfer to other specialist units if they need treatment for very specific difficulties. Transfer might occur directly from the neuro-rehabilitation centre, especially if the person requires assistance in managing specific problems, such as severe behavioural disturbance, which might be interfering with their progress in other areas. Neuro-rehabilitation may be resumed at a later stage when these issues are better managed.

Transfer to specialist placements

It is possible that your relative will not make the progress expected, will require additional specialist input, and that neither rehabilitation nor returning home will be viable options (see Chapter 2 on issues relating to recovery). In this event it is likely that they will be discharged to either a specialist long-term care and therapy unit or a nursing home (although these are not in plentiful supply). Patients who require this option usually have the following conditions.

Low-awareness states and persistent vegetative state

We have described these states in Chapter 2. If feeding is maintained and good nursing care is continued, a person can continue to live for many months or even years in such a condition. Life expectancy is reduced, mainly due to chest infections.

While occasional recovery from these states does occur, it is not common, and predicting who might recover and to what level is not possible, particularly in the first months after injury.

The treatment of a person in a vegetative state focuses on keeping him/her alive and on preventing complications. If the unresponsiveness lasts for several weeks, people often have a PEG (percutaneous endoscopic gastrostomy) tube inserted surgically through the skin directly into the stomach. In this way, a person can be fed over a long time. Nurses reposition the patient regularly to avoid pressure sores. Physiotherapists move the patient's arms and legs to keep them supple.

Families often benefit from longer-term emotional support in coming to terms with having a relative with such a condition.

Behavioural problems

A small number of individuals with persisting severe behavioural problems, in particular physical violence, may need long-term support and care in a specialist unit with a very tightly structured timetable.

The decision whether to place your relative in such a facility will need to be discussed very carefully with you and your relative as this can be a difficult time emotionally. Most family members do not wish this for their relative and can feel immense guilt. As well as securing emotional support for yourself, it is important to gather as much information about the residential options available; it may be necessary to visit/consider facilities that are a little further geographically from you to find something suitable for your relative. At this stage, families may find themselves in a 'limbo' type state—unsure if their relative will recover further.

A small number of patients may need to be transferred to specialist orthopaedic or spinal injury rehabilitation services instead of or as well as receiving neuro-rehabilitation services if they have extensive physical problems alongside the brain injury.

Availability of specialist rehabilitation services

All the rehabilitation services described are in short supply (a fact acknowledged by recent practice guidelines) so relatively few people can access them and usually only after a considerable waiting period. Specialist head injury services are also geographically disparate (with nothing in more rural areas), so you may need to be prepared to advocate actively for services on behalf of your relative, or to access those that are further afield. The national Headway helpline can be a useful source of information. In addition, your local Headway group may be able to provide information and support with this.

The vast majority of people with head injury are discharged home from hospital without further input. There are several reasons why this might occur: they may not have significant enough problems that require input, or they may not be deemed 'ready' for a period of intensive rehabilitation and require further time to recover physically (e.g. they may still be a little too unwell or tire too easily to be able to manage intensive therapy sessions). However, for many, despite an identified need for rehabilitation, there are few or no resources available in their locality.

Discharge home

The vast majority of people who sustain a head injury will be discharged home after initial hospital treatment, and only a handful of these will (for many reasons) go on to receive additional input after this. This transition home can be a worrying time for families and it is important to collect as much information as possible about what is available to you locally. Headway can be a good initial contact.

Sometimes the individual may have to leave the acute ward before a rehabilitation place is available, which can be a source of great family worry and stress, so it is important to get information about possible interim care arrangements. If they are to be discharged home first, it will be useful (and sometimes essential) to have your home assessed by an occupational therapist and physiotherapist (this is often called an access visit). This will address key issues such as the accessibility of your home, and the adequacy and safety of facilities for using the toilet, bathing, and so on.

It is also important to ensure that any practical help you will need (e.g. professional carers) is arranged. When your relative returns home, other family members may become involved in aspects of physical care (such as washing and dressing). This is fine as long as it is what you all want to happen—and this should be discussed with you before leaving home or the rehabilitation unit. If you do not want this (or after your relative returns home you find it too tiring or difficult) then you should think about accessing more formal help. This usually means contacting a care agency who employ trained carers to work with people in their own homes on a regular basis. The weekly plan of how many carers and when they visit is often referred to as a 'care package'. Social services can discuss with you how this can be organized and paid for (a care manager or social worker is usually central to this). They will usually need to assess the family finances as part of this process, so making time to gather together any financial paperwork can be helpful. The Citizen's Advice Bureau can provide advice on this. The telephone number for the social services departments for your area is listed in the telephone directory.

For most individuals who have been discharged home from hospital, initial symptoms and complaints such as headache, dizziness, and fatigue improve within days or weeks, although sometimes it takes months. Some symptoms may persist longer; they will be discussed in the following chapters. The injured person may experience very subtle problems (e.g. with concentration), and feel more irritable or low in mood. The irritability, sometimes leading to angry outbursts over little things, can be the most noticeable ongoing problem for the family. This is particularly troublesome if the injured person is not aware of their behaviour and denies that anything is wrong. Things that may help your relative at this stage include:

- encouraging them to rest regularly (and not rush back to work and other duties)
- reducing noise and other distractions at home (e.g. they may feel overwhelmed by lots of visitors).

Sometimes, headache and sleepiness become worse in the days after discharge. This does not necessarily indicate any danger, but occasionally it might be a sign that a subdural or extradural haematoma (bleeding inside the skull which compresses the brain (see Chapter 2)) is developing. Therefore a doctor should be consulted as soon as possible—either your GP or at the nearest A&E department. The doctor will do a clinical examination and possibly arrange a CT scan of the brain.

There are instances when injuries to other parts of the body are so severe that the head injury is not noticed in hospital. These patients may be discharged home after the fractures have been treated, and only when they try to return to work does it become evident that something is wrong with their memory or their behaviour. Also, other more subtle injuries become apparent only later, such as loss of smell and damage to the vestibular system in the inner ear, causing dizziness.

Discharge home with further neuro-rehabilitation input

Input on an outpatient basis can range from a follow-up by a doctor in a hospital outpatient clinic to outpatient therapy from rehabilitation professionals. Some hospitals make referrals to community rehabilitation teams who visit your relative at home; others make referrals to self-help organizations, such as Headway, or other specialist services (such as vocational rehabilitation schemes to support someone returning to work) if they exist in that area.

If your relative was previously receiving inpatient rehabilitation, the biggest issue for you all is likely to be adjustment to the reduction in the amount of therapy they will receive as an out-patient. It is likely to be of a much lower frequency than previously. This can cause distress and fear for patients and their relatives, as they worry that this will slow their recovery.

Discharge home without further input

The vast majority of people who have been seen in hospital for a head injury will be discharged home without further input. However, UK guidelines on the management of head injury highlight the need for all people presenting to A&E

departments with head injury to be given information about what possible complications can be expected, and how and when to seek further advice.

The guidelines also acknowledge that high levels of disability are experienced by large numbers of people after head injury, but that specialist services are sparse and geographically disparate. Thus there is a huge shortfall in the availability of services for those who need ongoing input.

Contact your GP in the first instance if you feel that your relative should be receiving these services but is currently not doing so.

When return home is not possible

Unfortunately, some patients will be unable to return home because it is unsafe for them to do so and they need higher levels of supervision or care than that which can be provided within their home environment. For example, an individual may have significant memory problems and need support with many aspects of everyday life. In these cases the level of care required exceeds the type of 'care package' described earlier and the best option is residential or nursing care placement. It is important that you are fully informed of all options and visit potential placements if possible. Funding for such placements can be complex and will depend on your relative's particular pattern of needs. Again, social services and the health professionals involved in your relative's care can advise you about this and provide information on available placements.

> In the UK there are now national guidelines commissioned by the NHS and health-professional groups which describe what should be available to you and your relative. These are listed at the end of this book. If you are unsure what sort of help your head-injured relative should be having at any stage or how help can be organized, ask your GP. If he/she is not sure, you may find Headway a useful place to start.

Recovery after head injury

In the previous chapter we started to discuss the important issue of recovery after head injury. Understandably this is one of the most important issues when a relative is injured and, unfortunately, one of the most difficult to address with any certainty.

While your relative is following the various pathways through different services and treatment teams in hospital and after discharge, the recovery process is taking place.

Mechanisms of recovery

How the brain 'recovers' after head injury is not fully understood. We know that it reacts to the damage by activating its repair systems. The blood from the haematomas and the 'debris' from the destroyed brain cells are cleaned up by the body's normal mechanisms. The oedema also drains away as the excess water is taken back into the blood stream. Unfortunately, unlike other parts of the body such as skin or bones, the brain is not good at regrowing those parts that have been irreversibly damaged. However, a few different processes in the brain do come into play that allow for some recovery. They are summarized under the term **plasticity** of the brain.

- Some brain cells have been temporarily damaged/injured, but not killed, and start to recover. It is thought that this can explain some of the initial improvement seen.

- Some neurons that have survived but lost their axons (their branches) can regrow them, thereby re-establishing contact with other brain cells by forming new connections (a kind of brain 'rewiring').

- In time, undamaged parts of the brain can learn to take over some of the functions of the damaged parts of the brain.

These processes are the basis of the spontaneous improvements that you witness in your relative's responsiveness and alertness, and in areas such as speech, memory, and movements.

'When will my relative get better?' or 'Will he/she make a full recovery?'

It is unfortunate that these most burning questions are the hardest for hospital staff to answer. If the doctors reply to you: 'We don't know yet. We will have to wait and see', they are being neither evasive nor incompetent. They are merely being honest and ensuring that they do not give you inaccurate information.

The rate and degree of recovery

The rate of recovery after head injury is as individual as each head injury, and therefore predictions are nearly impossible to make in the early stages. However, some general points about recovery can be applied to the 'average' person. There are several criteria that can be used to narrow down the possible future outcomes.

- The severity of the head injury is the best predictor of recovery. The more severe the injury, the longer is the recovery (and less recovery is usually made). However, there are always exceptions to this. Severity can be measured by the Glasgow Coma Scale (GCS), the length of post-traumatic amnesia (PTA), or the length of the person's unconsciousness (as described in Chapter 2).

- Age is a factor, as younger people have a better chance of a good recovery than the elderly.

- The location of the injury in the brain, as shown on the CT scan, determines the type of ongoing problems your relative may experience. This is because, as we saw in Chapter 2, different parts of the brain are specialized to perform certain functions, such as moving the arms and legs, speaking, or remembering.

- Quality of hospital care and treatment in the early stages.
- Availability of specialist rehabilitation.
- Support from family and friends.

Depending on these factors, any outcome is possible, from complete recovery (in most patients with mild head injury and some patients with moderate head injury) to early death or persistent vegetative state. Most people with moderate and severe head injury will not make a full recovery, but will retain some problems in one or more areas. These types of enduring problems are discussed in more detail in the following chapters.

When a person comes out of coma following a head injury, the first signs of recovery may appear in different ways, depending on which part of the brain was most severely damaged. Some people may start by saying a word in a slurred voice, others begin moving an arm or a leg, or they may open their eyes and look around the room. With ongoing improvement in levels of alertness, areas of particular difficulty become clearer. For instance, some patients may start recognizing their family members, speaking, and remembering who visited them the day before, but cannot move their left arm and leg. Others may regain good movement of arms and legs and start walking around, but are confused, restless, and agitated, and unable to tell who their family members are.

The recovery of a person after head injury is a gradual process which can take hours (in very mild cases only), but more likely days, weeks, months, or even years. It is never sudden. If your relative has been in a coma for a few days or longer, do not expect him/her to wake up suddenly and talk to you as if nothing had happened. Such recoveries are seen in Hollywood films, but sadly not in real life.

Recovery after head injury is fastest in the first 6 months or so, and then gradually slows down. However, improvement can continue for several years. This means that it is important not to give up hope too early. If you are with your relative every day, you may find, after a while, that you no longer notice further improvement. If this is the case, ask other relatives, friends, or medical professionals who only see your relative from time to time. Sometimes they are aware of positive changes that have occurred between visits which you had not noticed, because they have happened so slowly.

The term 'plateauing' is often used to describe the slowing down of recovery and is often synonymous with the ending of rehabilitation. Therefore this can be a time of great distress for patients and families. However, a slowing down of recovery does not necessarily imply a stopping of recovery; changes may occur sporadically, and improvements can be seen in people many years after injury. This can occur particularly if the person is offered further opportunities to learn alternative ways of managing or compensating for problems.

 Frequently asked questions

How long can we expect recovery to continue?

Recovery after head injury is fastest in the first 6 months or so, and it gradually slows down afterwards. However, improvement can continue for several years, particularly in people under 60 years of age. This means that you and your relative should not give up hope too early.

Is there anything we can do to speed up my relative's recovery?

Specialist rehabilitation is the only thing that has been shown to maximize the recovery of a person after head injury. So far, no drug has been found which is of benefit in speeding up the progress.

Would more therapy help?

Patients with moderate or severe head injury who have recovered to such an extent that they can actively participate in rehabilitation should have therapies on every working day. However, it must be realized that these patients fatigue easily, and therefore need rest periods in between therapy sessions. Having too much therapy can be just as detrimental as not getting enough.

Would a longer rehabilitation stay help?

Rehabilitation of patients after moderate or severe head injury in a specialist centre often lasts for several months. At some point, the advantages of therapies in the protected, but artificial, environment of the rehabilitation centre against the advantages of the patient returning to his/her familiar surrounding must be weighed up. Therefore longer does not automatically mean better.

4

Changes in physical functioning

⮊ Key points

◆ After a severe head injury, motor symptoms, swallowing deficits, sensory deficits, epileptic seizures, and loss of bladder and bowel control are common.

◆ Dizziness, headaches, and fatigue can occur not only after severe head injury, but also after mild head injury.

◆ Treatments which can help speed up recovery exist for most of these symptoms.

◆ Research has shown that families can cope well with their relative's physical changes when given advice and support.

In this chapter we focus on the physical problems that arise directly from injuries to those areas of the brain that are involved in movement control, balance, and processing of incoming information from the senses.

Motor/movement problems

Our movements are orchestrated by the brain in a highly complex manner which is usually quite reliable. This is achieved by a sophisticated interaction of several diverse centres in the brain. Each centre is specialized to a certain aspect of our movements: to keep us upright, to walk automatically, to start a movement, to stop it, to move powerfully or gently, or smoothly rather than jerkily.

After severe head injury, difficulties with moving different body parts are frequently found because of damage to areas such as the cerebellum and the motor cortex, leading to weakness, spasticity of limbs, reduced balance/coordination, and involuntary movements.

Muscle weakness

The most common motor problem is muscle weakness (**paresis**). It can be caused by damage to the parts of the brain which control our movements (e.g. the motor cortex) or by damage to the pathways through which nerve impulses from these centres are normally sent downwards to the spinal cord. Muscle weakness can occur in different patterns.

- **Hemiparesis** means that the injured person has a weakness on one side of his/her body: the arm, the leg, and sometimes the face is weak on the same side. Remember that left-sided weakness arises from right-sided brain injury, and vice versa. If this weakness is very severe, without any activity or movement, it is called **hemiplegia**.

- **Tetraparesis** (or quadriparesis) is the state in which an individual has weakness in all four limbs.

- **Paraparesis** means weakness in both legs. This can occur when the person has a spinal cord injury in addition to the head injury.

Weakness is typically worse in the hand than in the shoulder, and in the foot than in the hip. This is because separate parts of the brain are dedicated to controlling the muscles of the trunk and close to the trunk that keep us upright during sitting, standing, and walking. Sometimes these trunk muscles are also affected, particularly in the early stages after the injury. The patient may have difficulty sitting and keeping his/her head upright, and may need supporting by a person or something to lean on, such as pillows.

Recovery from muscle weakness is always gradual, not sudden, and it usually moves outwards from the trunk: the strength of the trunk improves before the strength of the arms and legs, and the strength of the hands and feet returns last.

Spasticity

In the days and weeks following the head injury, the paretic (weak) limbs sometimes become stiffer; when you try to move them, you can feel a resistance and the injured person can feel pain. This stiffness is called increased muscle tone or **spasticity**. It can occur in different patterns and you might hear your relative's doctor or physiotherapist use special terms to describe these patterns of stiffness. Typically after head injury, the spastic arm is **adducted** (pulled towards the trunk in the shoulder joint), the elbow, wrist, and fingers are **flexed** (bent), whereas the leg is mostly **extended** (straightened) in the knee, and the foot is **plantarflexed** (pointing downward) and **inverted** (pointing inward). Sometimes a spastic leg suddenly jumps (**spasm**), and it can shake rhythmically (**clonus**). Spasticity interferes with an individual's attempts to move his/her limbs and can lead to abnormal posture of arms, legs, or body. It can result in clumsiness and cause people to tire quickly. It adds yet another obstacle that has to be overcome during recovery.

Contractures

If a weak arm or leg is not moved regularly, an additional type of stiffness, called contracture, can develop in the soft tissues around the joints. This is caused by shortening of muscle fibres and development of fibrous tissue in the surrounding soft tissues. It is important to work hard to prevent this through exercise, because once contractures have developed, they can only be reversed by surgery.

Ataxia

Ataxia is a motor difficulty whereby the muscle power can be good, but the arm or leg performs jerky, clumsy, and uncoordinated movements. It is usually caused by damage to the cerebellum. Ataxia is often accompanied by limb **tremor** (rhythmic shaking).

Apraxia

Some patients have difficulty performing voluntary movements or actions (such as waving goodbye) because of a condition called **apraxia**. Here, patients do not necessarily have weakness or clumsiness in their movements, but the mental plan to perform a certain movement is disrupted. For instance, someone with this condition may be able to make a fist with full force, but when you ask them to act as if they were brushing their teeth, they cannot do it.

The **gait** (walking) is usually disturbed in patients with weakness or ataxia of one or both legs, making them insecure on their legs. If they try to stand up and walk without help, they are at great risk of falling and injuring themselves.

Ways to help your relative with motor problems

Physical difficulties are likely to cause your relative and yourself a great deal of concern. Being unable to walk, sit unaided, control fine motor movements, and so on will obviously have an impact on the person's ability to return to their previous roles and responsibilities (care for themselves, return to work, driving, etc.). The pattern/types of physical difficulties your relative experiences after their head injury will be unique to them. What follows is an overview of some of the treatments on offer. Further information and support can be found in Appendix 1.

Physiotherapy

Some physical difficulties can be treated by physiotherapy. Physiotherapists employ therapies to improve muscle control of the whole body, balance, and walking. They:

- help the individual rebuild their strength
- refine their coordination
- improve their posture and gait
- reduce spasticity
- alleviate pain
- prevent complications such as contractures.

Active physiotherapy

The patient is encouraged to perform activities, and the therapist gives feedback to help them achieve fine control of specific muscles. At first, the individual may only be able to lift the arm in the shoulder joint. The movement is practised, and if recovery of muscles of the upper arm and forearm begins, this will be incorporated into the exercises. Exercises steadily become more difficult. The same is true for recovery of motor function of the legs: the patient will practise standing before he/she starts walking. Therapists will aim to help the individual perform the movements in a manner that is as close as possible to the normal healthy way. This is not always achievable if the injury has damaged the motor areas of the brain so severely (see Chapter 2) that the arm or leg does not regain **its former strength. In this case, the therapist will work with the patient to practise** and learn alternative ways of achieving the goal.

Passive therapy

This counters the effect of spasticity by relaxing tight muscles. It includes lying the patient on his/her side, or sitting or standing him/her in a support frame and performing gentle stretching exercises. You may be asked to do these with your relative following discharge from the rehabilitation centre, once you have been trained by the physiotherapists.

Putting a spastic limb in a plaster cast can prolong the stretching effect and helps to achieve a more natural position. Adaptive equipment and mobility aids include:

* ankle–foot orthoses (AFOs)—foot splints made from plastic—to keep the foot at an angle of 90° during walking

* arm or leg splints to support weak muscles or counter spasticity

* canes and frames (e.g. a Zimmer frame) to aid walking.

The therapist will train your relative how and when to use these. Your relative may be advised to use a wheelchair even if he/she has started to walk again, either to help conserve energy or to remain safe if there are problems with balance. An occupational therapist will advise on what sort of wheelchair would be most suitable for your relative. This may need to be reviewed over time if your relative's movement abilities or needs change significantly.

Other treatments

Additional therapeutic techniques can be used in conjunction with the methods described above.

* **Hydrotherapy** is physiotherapy performed in a swimming pool.

* **Treadmill training** with partial body-weight support is a technique in which the patient is strapped into a harness hanging above a treadmill on which he/she practises walking.

- **Constraint-induced movement therapy**, also called forced-use therapy, immobilizes the patient's unaffected arm in a sling or a splint for several hours a day, forcing him/her to use the affected arm for all activities.

- **Functional electrical stimulation** (**FES**) elicits muscle contractions with electric impulses.

Specific treatments to reduce spasticity include drugs such as baclofen, tizanidine, or gabapentin (which are taken by mouth), and injections with botulinum toxin. In severe cases, **surgical treatments** such as the implantation of a baclofen pump or lengthening of muscles or tendons can be considered.

How to support your relative with mobility problems

If your relative is not accessing physiotherapy but is experiencing any of the problems described, you should seek advice from your GP or organizations such as Headway. If your relative is undertaking rehabilitation you might find it helpful to attend sessions as well, to see how they have been taught and how you can help safely. In addition, your relative may find your presence reassuring.

> Be patient and avoid doing things for your relative if they can and want to do things for themselves, even if it takes longer. They are more likely to get faster as well as feel much better if they manage to complete tasks themselves.

It can help to be aware that people with head injury can experience high levels of anxiety (about issues such as falling, or about whether they will recover fully) and these concerns can interfere with their confidence when working on physical problems. Ask for help if your relative's worries do not respond to support and reassurance.

One of the most important ways that you can help your relative is to collect all available information and be aware of what services are available in their area and how to access them.

- Make sure that you show as much understanding as possible of any physical problems and the best ways to get around them and stop them getting worse.

- If your relative agrees, make sure that you ask their GP or other professionals questions at every opportunity about what you can do to help.

- Try to make sure that you both have all the necessary information and advice before buying any expensive equipment or planning expensive alterations to your home.

Swallowing problems

Swallowing problems are common after head injury (i.e. to be able to eat and drink without the risk of food or liquids going down the wrong way onto the lungs, which could result in choking and/or chest infection). As with most problems after head injury, the nature and severity of these difficulties will depend on the location and extent of damage to the brain. Problems with swallowing are caused by weakness of, or difficulty in coordinating the muscles involved in swallowing as well as control of breathing.

People with head injury may be able to swallow saliva but be unsafe to eat or drink other types of fluid or foods. Less severe, but very troublesome, can be problems with drooling/dribbling of saliva which can cause social embarrassment. If a person is thought to have swallowing difficulties they will be referred to a speech and language therapist (SALT) for assessment of their swallowing (this might occur in a hospital setting or in the community).

The SALT will advise on whether the person is safe to eat and drink or not, and whether any modifications are needed to the consistency of food and drink given to make it safe for the individual. For example, sometimes fluids should be thickened using a drink-thickening powder which will be prescribed. They will recommend the consistency, e.g. to the consistency of single cream or syrup, to make them safer to swallow. It is important that advice from a SALT is taken before attempting to thicken fluids yourself. They will also advise on positions to make swallowing safer (e.g. sitting upright with chin tucked slightly down to swallow). Many people do not enjoy having an adapted diet of thickened liquids and/or pureed food, and this can be a source of tension within families, with meal times losing their enjoyment and pleasure for the injured person.

Most swallowing problems can be assessed and diagnosed by clinical examination and oral trials by a SALT. However, additional examinations might include the following.

- **Fibre-optic endoscopic evaluation of swallowing** (**FEES**) A camera is passed up the patient's nose and into their throat to observe muscle movement and residue post-swallow.

- **Videofluoroscopy** A moving X-ray where a person is asked to swallow some radio-opaque mixture mixed into different food textures and consistencies to assess the safety of their swallowing and the impact of various strategies.

If the person is unsafe to eat or drink, i.e. there is a risk of food or drink going down the wrong way into their lungs (**aspiration**), non-oral feeding (i.e. feeding via a tube not via the mouth) will be advised. Aspiration can cause severe chest infections. Non-oral feeding may initially be intravenous and then a **nasogastric tube** (a tube up the nose and down to the stomach) may be passed to allow special liquid feed and fluids to be given non-orally. For persistent problems with swallowing it may be recommended that a **percutaneous endoscopic gastrostomy (PEG)** tube be inserted throught the abdominal wall into the stomach to enable feeding. The decision as to which method is used will be made by the doctor in charge of the person's care, following advice from the dietician, the SALT, and nurses, and discussion with the patient and their family as appropriate.

As the person's swallowing improves, eating and drinking will be started under supervision. The PEG tube does not prevent someone from starting to eat or drink when it is safe, and the tube can be removed once it is no longer required.

Sensory problems after head injury

If a person has mobility problems after a head injury, he/she usually also has sensory loss in the same arm and leg. This is because the centres of the brain which control movements and those which control sensation are very close together. Having less sensation in a hand or foot means that the person does not feel objects in their hand properly, and cannot feel the floor underfoot as usual. Therefore reduced sensation has a negative impact on moving the arm and on walking safely. Patients who have lost the ability to distinguish hot and cold are at risk of burning themselves.

Managing loss of sensation

Sensation which has been lost may gradually improve, but it cannot be restored by therapies or exercises in the same way that motor loss can. Treatment of sensory loss consists mainly of reminding the patient to pay attention to where they put their hand or foot. By concentrating on the movements, they will gradually become more precise. This is something that you can help your relative with.

Visual deficits

Problems with vision can manifest themselves in different ways, depending on the site of the brain injury.

Loss of vision in one eye can occur as a consequence of injury to the eye, or the optic nerve which transports the visual information from the eye into the brain. The severity of loss of vision may range from mildly blurred vision in the affected eye to complete blindness of the eye.

Visual field defects in both eyes are usually caused by damage to the brain, not the eye. In these cases, patients cannot see what is on one side of their visual fields of both eyes: either on the right side in both eyes or the left side in both eyes. This visual deficit is called **hemianopia**. These patients sometimes bump into door frames or people on their left or right sides because they cannot see them. Hemianopia needs to be distinguished from a condition called **hemineglect**

where the individual is not aware of one side (mostly the left side) of the space around them and their own body.

Double vision occurs when the coordination of the movement of both eyes is disrupted, and the eyes move independently of each other.

Managing visual deficits

Visual problems after head injury can be very debilitating and distressing and, if not dealt with, can hinder your relative's progress in other areas of their recovery. The first step in helping the individual to cope with a visual deficit is to diagnose the precise nature of the problem by a test in the eye hospital where ophthalmologists can prescribe visual aids, such as glasses, or an eye patch in the case of double vision. There are no visual aids available to improve hemianopia, but patients usually learn to compensate for the defect by scanning with their eyes towards the blind side. The rehabilitation team can train them in achieving this.

Hearing disturbance

Injury to the outer or inner ear can cause hearing loss on one or both sides. In some cases, people develop **tinnitus**, an unpleasant ringing in one ear. The treatment for hearing loss is a hearing aid, but there is no rehabilitation technique to train the deaf ear to hear better. There is no medical treatment for tinnitus, but psychological therapies can be helpful in assisting people to learn to live with it.

Loss of smell

This occurs quite frequently after head injury, but it is often not noticed right away. It may become obvious when a person with head injury puts on too much aftershave or perfume, or they do not smell food burning on the cooker. No treatment exists to improve sense of smell, and so the patient needs to be encouraged to check food that is cooking and possibly adapt their environment to increase their safety, such as having smoke detectors installed. Often, improvement occurs spontaneously, but it can take a long time.

Dizziness and balance problems

The inner ear contains the vestibular system which helps us keep our equilibrium or balance. It tells us which position our head is in, or which way we are turning our head, even with our eyes closed. If the vestibular system is damaged, people suffer from dizziness and problems with balance. Moving the head, bending over, riding bicycles, and other movements make the dizziness worse and can cause nausea. The vestibular system is so delicate that it can be damaged even in a minor head injury. A doctor can diagnose damage to the vestibular system by observing the patient's eyes closely: sometimes a fine shaking of the eyes, called **nystagmus,** can be seen.

Dizziness is not easy to treat. Vestibular rehabilitation with balance retraining exercises can be taught by a physiotherapist, and drugs such as prochlorperazine may help if the dizziness is accompanied by nausea. Frequently, however, individuals who suffer from dizziness will have to be supported to learn to live with it and continue with their daily life, which they are mostly able to do over time. Sometimes, dizziness is a side effect of medication, in which case the drug should be replaced with another one. Dizziness can also result from, or be made worse by, the emotional stress associated with having had the head injury.

Pain and headache

Headache and other pain conditions (particularly neck pain) are frequent after severe head injury, but can also occur after mild head injury. Usually, pain diminishes slowly over time. Sometimes the pain is caused by injury to the muscles and tendons in the neck. If the pain arises from the neck, physiotherapy, which can include training of posture, massage, and hot/cold packs, often helps. Otherwise, drug treatment with pain killers such as aspirin or paracetamol is sometimes necessary.

In other cases, the headaches appear like migraine attacks triggered by the head injury. Visual problems can also cause headache. If the headache has features of migraine, then the GP may decide to prescribe migraine medication. If the pain persists over a longer period of time, psychological therapies can be helpful.

Fatigue

After head injury, many patients feel less fit, have reduced stamina, and get tired easily after even small exertions. This is common after all head injuries and can have several causes, the most important being a diffuse axonal injury (see Chapter 2) which causes communication between different brain centres to be disrupted and slow down to some extent. Consequently every physical or mental activity requires extra effort and extra concentration and therefore is exhausting. Mood disturbances such as depression or anxiety can also contribute to the fatigue.

Fatigue can have a major impact on family life. In addition to restricting activities, it can also lead to increased feelings of frustration and irritability for the person who is fatigued. Learning to manage fatigue and reduce its effect on everyday life is a real skill. It often involves the individual relearning how to spend his/her time each day and how to approach tasks. Key aspects of fatigue management include learning to rest regularly and pacing yourself. If fatigue is a problem for your relative, it is helpful to gain more information about how (and when) this is affecting them. Simply observing their behaviour may also give you important clues. You should raise this with the professionals involved in their care (or their GP if they are not accessing rehabilitation). They can provide your relative with more advice and support in dealing with this.

Epileptic seizures

When the brain has been injured, repair mechanisms clean up the debris from the destroyed brain cells, but a scar remains in place where the brain has lost its well-organized structure. In these scarred areas, brain cells can become over-excited and generate electric impulses which are spread throughout the brain within seconds. This results in the individual having a seizure, 'fit', or convulsion. This is sometimes referred to as **post-traumatic epilepsy**.

Epileptic seizures can manifest themselves in a variety of ways.

- **Grand mal seizures** (or tonic–clonic seizures) are the most widely known. The person loses consciousness and falls to the ground, the body stiffens up, and both arms and legs go into violent shakes. Sometimes the sufferer bites their tongue or the inside of their cheeks, and sometimes they lose urine or lose control of their bowels. In most cases, the seizures end by themselves within a few minutes. Afterwards, a person is typically very tired for the rest of the day and has no recollection of anything that happened during the seizure.

- **Complex focal seizures** (or complex partial seizures) are sometimes incorrectly referred to as 'absences'. Here, the individual suddenly stops talking or whatever they were doing and stares into the air. Sometimes they do strange things such as grimacing or pulling on their clothes. Usually they are not aware of what is happening, and they do not respond when spoken to. Unlike grand mal seizures, consciousness is not lost completely, but it is disturbed to some degree. In most instances these seizures last less than a minute, and the person does not remember them.

- **Simple focal seizures** (or simple partial seizures): consciousness is neither completely lost (as in the grand mal seizure) nor even disturbed (as during the complex focal seizure). The affected person may develop rhythmic shaking of an arm or a leg or both, experience strange sensations in these limbs, or twitching of the corner of the mouth. They are fully aware of what is happening to them, and they remember it afterwards.

Sometimes a simple or complex focal seizure turns into a grand mal seizure.

In the first days after a severe head injury, epileptic seizures are common, particularly after penetrating head injuries (see Chapter 2). Therefore it is common practice to start patients on anti-convulsant drugs such as phenytoin to prevent future seizures. Because seizures are so common in this situation, patients are not diagnosed with epilepsy unless seizures recur after weeks or months. The risk of having a seizure gradually decreases the longer the individual remains seizure free. Unfortunately, however, even patients who were initially free of fits can have their first seizure months or even years after the injury.

Epilepsy is a frightening condition for the patient and distressing for family and others to observe, particularly when it happens for the first time. In most cases, seizures occur without warning and can result in serious injuries. Occasionally patients experience an 'aura' beforehand—an unusual and strange feeling which can provide some warning. Despite the unpredictability of epileptic seizures, many epilepsy sufferers lead quite normal lives and succeed in holding onto a job. Driving a car is not allowed for a year following each seizure, even 'small' simple focal seizures.

There are a number of well-known triggers which can bring about an epileptic seizure, and which should therefore be avoided:

- lack of sleep
- flickering light
- psychological stress
- alcohol
- some drugs, such as certain antibiotics.

If a person is suspected of having epileptic seizures, an **electroencephalogram (EEG)** can be performed in which the electrical activity of the brain is measured with electrodes on the surface of the skull. If the EEG shows typical spike–wave patterns, epilepsy is confirmed. Unfortunately, a normal EEG does not exclude epilepsy, as people with epilepsy can have normal EEG periods between seizures.

The treatment of epilepsy is based on avoiding the triggers and taking anti-epileptic medication. Frequently used drugs are phenytoin, carbamazepine, and lamotrigine. With these drugs, many patients remain seizure free, but may experience side effects such as sleepiness, drowsiness, and eczema. Once an individual has been on anti-epileptic drugs, they should never stop taking them abruptly, as this greatly increases the risk of having a seizure. If someone has remained seizure free for a long time, they should discuss with their neurologist whether it is safe to reduce the dose.

Supporting your relative who has epilepsy

When you witness a person having a seizure, particularly if it is a grand mal seizure, the most important thing to do is to ensure that the individual is safe. Most epileptic seizures terminate by themselves within a minute or two. If the seizure happens at home, you do not need to call an ambulance unless the seizure continues for more than 5 minutes. Discuss with the doctor who is in charge of your relative's epilepsy treatment whether you should carry midazolam liquid with you. This drug can be squirted into the patient's mouth to stop the seizure.

Bladder and bowel problems

After head injury some patients have difficulty controlling their bladder and bowels. This is called **incontinence** and is obviously an embarrassing condition, for which your relative requires understanding and reassurance from you.

If the problem is only mild, with the occasional incontinence of urine, a medication such as oxybutynin may help. If the problem is more severe, a urinary catheter can be inserted through the urethra into the bladder, allowing the urine to flow into a bag. These catheters can cause bladder infections. If the incontinence persists, suprapubic catheters can be used which are inserted surgically through the abdominal wall into the bladder. Alternatives are catheters that are attached to a condom, or incontinence pads. In order to help your relative to achieve continence, the nurses will try to establish a more regular toileting routine with them. Once your relative has returned home, both of you will need to decide whether you will be the one to help with the toileting, or whether it should be done by professional carers. Simple changes to your relative's environment may also help to reduce the impact of bladder problems, for example moving them to a bedroom that is nearer the lavatory, and making sure that they have urine bottles close to hand near the bed. Make sure that your relative knows where the nearest toilet is if they have problems with remembering. Your GP will be able to refer you to a community-based continence advisor who can support you and your relative with this problem.

How physical problems affect your relative's everyday life

The physical problems discussed in this chapter can, alone or in combination, make everyday life difficult.

Apparently simple acts such as dressing and washing, making a cup of tea, and going shopping can be difficult, slow, or impossible. Treatment for problems with self-care and other everyday activities is provided mainly by occupational therapists and nurses if your relative is participating in rehabilitation. In Chapter 3 we discussed compensatory techniques: they will often be used in dressing and washing practice when an individual has lost power in one arm and has to learn to do everything with the other arm or by using special aids (e.g. a long-handled brush). Activities such as making a cup of tea and going shopping are also the domain of the occupational therapists who practice them with your relative. The practice starts simply and is slowly made more and more difficult and complicated. This is very frustrating and means that your relative needs not only physical help, but also emotional support.

❓ Frequently asked questions

♦ **What about the use of alternative therapies, such as acupuncture, seeing a chiropractor, massage, etc.? Will they help my relative?**

There is insufficient evidence from clinical studies available to pass judgement on whether they are helpful or not. If your relative is considering any form of alternative therapy, it is useful to discuss this with their doctor or other professionals involved in their care in the first instance.

♦ **Is it safe for my relative to drink alcohol?**

After head injury, people typically do not tolerate alcohol very well. This means that they can get drunk more easily, which may affect not only their behaviour towards others, but also their movements—they can fall over more readily. Therefore it is recommended they drink alcohol in moderation only. If your relative is on anti-epileptic medication, he/she should drink as little as possible. Alcohol increases the risk of epileptic seizures, and both alcohol and drugs are a burden on the liver.

♦ **My relative has difficulty swallowing. Will he/she be able to eat and drink again?**

This depends on the nature and severity of the swallowing problem. Following assessment, the speech and language therapist (SALT) will usually be able to advise on whether the swallowing problem is likely to be long term. Often time will tell, and a person's swallow may sometimes improve long after injury.

♦ **Will he/she be able to eat normal food again?**

Commonly, the recovery of a swallowing problem is gradual. When the team feel that it is safe to begin eating and drinking, food will be introduced gradually and cautiously, often starting with a specific food consistency only.

5

Changes in thinking skills

→ Key points

- Cognitive (thinking) difficulties after a head injury are common.
- Cognitive changes, even if mild, can have a major impact on everyday life.
- The nature and extent of cognitive difficulties will depend on how severe the injury is and the brain areas damaged.
- Cognitive problems are associated with poorer long-term outcomes such as failure to return to work.
- Although challenging and stressful, the impact of cognitive problems can be minimized by:
  - making changes to the environment
  - altering the demands placed on relative
  - using a range of simple aids.
- Professional support in this area can be accessed via GP and specialist services.

In this chapter we will look at the most common cognitive (thinking) problems that can occur after head injury, the causes of these, and what can be done about them. The key to coping with your relative's cognitive difficulties is to **become knowledgeable** about the problems that can occur, **use simple strategies** and **aids**, **alter your relative's home and work environment**, and learn to **look after yourself** and know what forms of emotional and practical support are available to you.

Cognition (or cognitive functioning) refers to the whole range of **thinking processes** that we all engage in. This umbrella term includes:

- our memory
- our ability to concentrate and pay attention to things
- multi-tasking
- being able to think quickly and flexibly

- recognizing objects and remembering their names and uses
- our ability to reason and solve problems
- being able to plan and organize what we do

Cognitive abilities are essential for everyday life—we constantly draw on all these aspects of thinking.

Common thinking problems after head injury: an overview

Changes in cognitive functioning frequently occur after a head injury. The nature and extent of your relative's cognitive difficulties will depend on how severe their injury is and the brain areas damaged.

Some thinking processes are associated with specific areas of the brain. Others involve different parts of the brain working together. Although every head injury is different, we know that particular brain areas are more vulnerable to damage. The common areas damaged after a head injury (see Chapter 2) make certain types of cognitive problems more likely. However, there are no hard and fast rules, and a range of other factors unique to your relative (such as their age, general health before the injury, and abilities in each of these areas before their injury) are also influential and mean that the picture seen after each head injury is different for everyone.

As we most commonly see damage to the frontal and temporal lobes, together with diffuse axonal injuries throughout the brain, typical problems are:

- slower thinking speed
- reduced flexibility in thinking
- difficulties with remembering and learning new information
- problems with attention and concentration
- poor planning and organizational skills
- poor reasoning and judgement.

We know that these types of cognitive changes have a much greater impact on long-term outcome (such as return to work) than physical problems. Families also tell us that these types of problems cause them the greatest confusion and distress.

Thinking problems and the severity of the head injury

The extent of cognitive or thinking difficulties depends to a large part on the severity of the head injury. Severity is classified by doctors according to the length of time that the individual is unconscious (GCS) and the time taken to become fully aware of their surroundings (PTA) (see Chapter 1).

Mild head injury

After even a mild head injury it is common for individuals to feel confused and disorientated. In the case of a very mild head injury these problems usually resolve quite quickly. In some cases, however, small cognitive changes do occur and these may endure over time. Although subtle, these can have a significant impact on everyday life, including work (especially if the person is returning to a demanding job) and family life. The danger is that these subtle problems may be overlooked because the individual seems to have made a full recovery. Problems may only emerge when they are faced with unfamiliar or complex tasks, or if they are tired or under stress. Such mild changes can still cause confusion and worry to individuals, and confidence levels can fall. The impact on other family members can also be significant.

More severe head injuries

If your relative has had a moderate or severe head injury, he/she is more likely to experience some degree of difficulty with thinking and memory. Although these may improve over time, long-lasting changes are much more frequently seen. Such difficulties can have a major impact on everyday life, restricting opportunities for returning to work, and can be difficult for families and the injured person to understand. As with minor injuries, the nature and extent of difficulties may not always be apparent until later—for example, when your relative tries to return to work.

Changes in memory abilities

Memory is an extremely complicated, and sometimes misunderstood, system. What we refer to as memory is actually made up of several subsystems, with different types of memory being organized in different brain areas. We have separate memory systems for different types of information, including:

- verbal information
- visual information
- personal events (i.e. what has happened to us throughout our lives)
- facts about the world/general knowledge
- our memory for skills (like driving and playing a musical instrument).

In addition to these subsystems, we have a temporary memory store which we use to hold information for very brief periods of time while we do something with it (e.g. write down a phone number), before it is forgotten or transferred to a more permanent store.

There are also different stages of memory, any of which can go wrong when memory is not working properly. First, in order to remember something at a later time we need to pay attention to it and process it in some way (this stage is called encoding and involves our temporary memory store), and then we need to rehearse it (repeat it or practice it) or make links with information we already have in memory in order to store it in our more permanent memory store (this is called consolidation), before finally getting it back out of our memory when we need it (retrieval).

Often people draw comparisons between memory and other complex storage systems (like a complicated filing system). It might help you to try and think about it as a filing cabinet. New memories may be stored initially for a brief period in the top drawer (like our temporary memory store) while waiting to be filed away properly (in the appropriate place with similar files). The process of filing it away properly in the right place is like the consolidation stage of memory. Later retrieval will depend on how good your filing system is. For your memory to work well, you need an efficient well-organized system, storing files on similar topics together.

How is memory typically affected after a head injury?

Although memory functioning often changes after a head injury, the way our memories are organized within our brains means that the entire memory system will not be affected. Someone would not typically lose all their memories and memory abilities. When we say that someone's memory is damaged after head injury, what we mean is that one (or more) *parts* of the memory system have become damaged. Others will be completely intact.

We explained in Chapter 2 how in the very early stages of recovery, it is common for individuals to experience post-traumatic amnesia (PTA). At this stage their ability to remember any new information may seem severely affected. This typically resolves over time (although the length of PTA does vary between individuals). However, when the period of PTA passes, there may be ongoing problems with memory, particularly if the head injury is severe. Typically, after a head injury, a person will have most difficulty with the following.

- ◆ **Learning and remembering new information** Generally, after head injury it becomes much more difficult to take on board new information and lay down new everyday memories. The injured individual may be unable to learn any new information, may only remember parts of it (their recall is patchy), or may find learning to be very slow and effortful. Thinking back to our filing cabinet example, the new files are not being properly stored—perhaps falling down the back of the top drawer, and never being put into the correct storage space. Generally, individuals tend to have better memory for things that happened before the accident (e.g. from their childhood).

- ◆ **'Remembering to remember'** This refers to our memory for things in the future (i.e. remembering to do something, like keep an appointment or complete a job that needs doing at a certain time). You might hear this referred to as prospective memory. This type of memory (which involves the frontal lobes) is obviously important in everyday life.

◆ **Remembering events leading up to the head injury** It is unusual for people to remember the events leading up to the head injury itself. This period of memory loss, referred to as **retrograde amnesia**, differs in length between individuals. It can range from a few minutes to hours, days, or even months before the injury occurred. Although this can improve over time, with individuals gradually regaining some memories, the memory of the event itself is never retrieved. Individuals are often preoccupied with this loss of memory and may be distressed by not remembering the event, despite it being traumatic in nature.

> Older memories, memories of general knowledge and facts, and memories of skills are usually relatively well preserved after head injury.

How are memory problems seen in everyday life?

Because of the complex nature of memory, how your relative comes across to you and others might sometimes seem contradictory or puzzling. Families often say that they have been struggling to understand why their relative remembers events from his/her distant past yet is unable to remember something he/she heard yesterday. Thinking back to our filing cabinet, imagine that the old memory files were well ordered previously and thus easy to find; in contrast, the newer files are being misplaced and never properly filed away.

Your relative may also seem very forgetful, for example forgetting to complete a job you have asked him/her to do. You might notice that your relative needs you to repeat information on several occasions and to give him/her frequent reminders, or they may need considerably more practice at doing something before it becomes routine. They may also lose their enjoyment of certain activities (e.g. reading the newspaper or watching a film) if they cannot remember what they have just read or seen. Consequently, they may find memory changes very frustrating, upsetting, and disruptive.

Memory also plays an important role in our sense of who we are and how we view ourselves. Our 'sense of self' depends on having intact and continuous personal memories—for example, remembering key events and achievements, such as the birth of children, throughout our lives. Being unable to remember this type of information, or having 'gaps' in our memories, makes it difficult to retain a clear picture in our minds of the type of person we are or how we have developed over time. This can be baffling and distressing.

Changes in thinking speed

Thinking speed, sometimes referred to as **information processing speed**, is the time it takes for us to process the everyday information that we see or hear, from initially registering it, to thinking it through, and then responding in some way.

Being able to think quickly depends on information being transmitted at speed along nerve fibres. After a head injury, the nerve pathways throughout the brain are disrupted and therefore messages take longer to get through. Therefore a slowdown in thinking speed is very common after a head injury (even after a mild one).

How is thinking speed typically affected after head injury?

You may find that, after a head injury your relative is unable to do things as quickly as previously. He/she may be unable to follow a conversation or to make a decision quickly. As a result of trying to 'keep up' it is typical for individuals to become 'mentally' overloaded quite quickly and to become irritable. You may notice that your relative loses his/her temper more easily, tires quickly, or ends tasks or conversations more suddenly than usual. He/she may be less able to cope with the demands and stresses placed on them.

Changes in this area can have a significant impact on the injured individual as it may mean that he/she is unable to return to work and family roles. Quick thinking is also essential in driving, and therefore reduced processing speed may restrict someone's ability to drive safely.

Changes in attention

Like memory, attention is a complex process. There are many different types of attention, or attention systems, which we use in everyday life including:

- concentrating for a long period of time (on a work assignment or when watching a film)
- multi-tasking
- concentrating hard on one thing if there are distractions around (e.g. 'tuning out' background noise from the TV while talking to someone).

The frontal lobes play an important role in all of the above. Particularly in the early stages of recovery, it is common to see difficulties with all these systems.

Changes in attention can also have a major impact on memory—it is difficult to learn and remember new information if you do not pay attention to it initially! In addition, we draw extensively on these abilities when we are carrying out complex tasks such as driving and in the work environment. Thus changes in this area can have a significant impact on the individual's ability to do these successfully.

How might attentional problems be seen in everyday life?

This will depend on what specific aspects of attention and concentration have been affected. If your relative has difficulties sustaining their attention, they may seem to daydream or drift off in the middle of a task, or they may be unable to follow a film. Their attention span may seem particularly short in the early stages—your relative may only be able to concentrate for a few minutes at a time.

It is also likely that your relative will find it much harder to cope with or tolerate distractions around them. You may notice that if someone walks into the room your relative becomes distracted, or they may be unable to cope with any background noise, losing the thread of their conversation if someone is talking in the background. Such difficulties are not restricted to noise only—individuals may have difficulty if there is a lot of visual 'clutter' (e.g. having difficulty focusing on or finding one thing if there is a lot to look at). In particular, they may find it hard to tolerate children. At such times, your relative may feel 'overloaded' by all the extra stimulation and noise they are unable to filter out and ignore. They may then become upset or irritable.

Before the head injury, your relative may have thought nothing of doing two (or more!) tasks at once—for example, preparing a meal while helping a child do homework. This can become impossible after a head injury.

Changes in 'executive abilities'

The front part of our brain, which is very susceptible to damage in a head injury, plays a key role in our most complex thinking processes. These include planning, reasoning things out, and getting started on tasks. It also influences our behaviour by controlling our impulses, and ensuring that it is appropriate to the situations in which we find ourselves. In fact, it oversees and organizes all our other cognitive functions and is often thought of as being similar to a chief executive in a company who takes responsibility for checking that everything is working satisfactorily (that is why these brain processes are sometimes referred to as executive processes). If this 'executive' is not working properly, we can see a range of problems. These include loss of flexibility in thinking, impaired initiation (difficulties getting started on things), impaired problem solving, an inability to break down complicated tasks into a clear sequence to work through, and changes in behaviour.

What problems in executive functioning are typically seen after head injury?

As a result of damage to the frontal lobes, the individual may experience problems in any of the 'higher-level' thinking processes outlined above. In particular, they may find it difficult to think things through logically and flexibly or be unable to plan and organize themselves and their work, problem-solve, and make sound judgements. They may also show changes in behaviour and personality—for example, individuals may be unable to stop themselves from saying or doing inappropriate things (e.g. swearing), or be unaware of their behaviour and its impact on other people.

How might executive problems be seen in everyday life?

Problems with higher-level thinking skills including

◆ **Perseveration** You may notice that your relative's thinking is quite 'concrete' in its style: this means that they may get stuck on one topic of conversation or task, even if what they are doing is not working for them (i.e. they persist with this and are unable to switch to a new topic or way of working). This is sometimes referred to as perseveration.

◆ **Planning and organizational difficulties** Individuals may also be at a loss when faced with new or unfamiliar tasks that require planning and organization. They may find that they get lost or confused when faced with a job that does not have much structure. Even tasks that were previously completed fairly easily (e.g. cooking a meal) can become very difficult as they require the individual to coordinate lots of different steps and timings. Such sequencing difficulties may also be seen on simple tasks if problems are severe.

◆ **Problem-solving difficulties** You may notice that your relative seems to manage tasks well until a problem is encountered, at which point they may find themselves stuck and unable to plan what to do next. These changes can be subtle and may not manifest themselves straight away.

◆ **Reduced initiation** This refers to a particular problem in starting tasks (e.g. a household chore). The problem does not lie in the task itself—people with reduced initiation can usually complete the task successfully once they have been encouraged to begin the first steps.

Behaviour and personality changes

We know that personality and behaviour changes are common after head injury and damage to the frontal lobes. Changes include:

◆ **disinhibition** (e.g. saying hurtful things, swearing, being unable to control angry impulses)

◆ **egocentricity** (becoming very focused on their own needs and unable to consider others)

◆ **impulsivity** (acting quickly and without full consideration of what the individual is about to do)

◆ **passivity** (e.g. becoming withdrawn; showing no emotional response).

We know that such changes are particularly upsetting for families, more than any other changes associated with head injury. These are outlined in more detail in Chapter 7: 'Changes in emotions and behaviour'.

Reduced awareness

Sometimes after a head injury, people show no or only very limited awareness (or insight) of their difficulties—for example, they may not recognize that they have memory problems, that their speech is unclear, or that they are unable to walk safely. This is not always an all-or-nothing phenomenon. Individuals may show awareness of some changes but not all. Consequently, their judgement may be poor and they may inadvertently place themselves in risky situations (e.g. trying to get back to driving).

Reduced insight means that your relative may not be aware of some of the changes that you, other relatives and friends, or professionals are noticing. For example, your relative might want to do something that you know they are currently unable to do (like make a hot drink or climb the stairs). Your attempts to protect them (whether from danger or simply failing on a task) may be misunderstood by them and taken as attempts to hold them back—this can lead to feelings of resentment and anger. Your relative may also have reduced insight into changes in their behaviour, thus creating some social difficulties and awkward social situations. This can be extremely distressing for all and a source of considerable tension within the family.

Reduced awareness or denial?

Changes in awareness are directly related to the brain injury itself and the areas of the brain affected (the frontal lobes). This is quite different from the more psychological phenomenon of denial. Denial is when the individual is aware of the changes experienced but does not want to admit to or think about them. Denial is not necessarily harmful. It can often be helpful in the short term as it may protect someone from becoming depressed or anxious, but in the longer term it may cause more problems. It is sometimes difficult to tease these two out. Sometimes the picture is even more complicated as the two can occur together.

Changes in visual perception

Perception refers to how the brain makes sense of information coming in through the senses. An uninjured brain is normally able to interpret accurately the visual information coming in from the eyes along the optic nerve. This information is used to make judgements about what we see—for example, to recognize objects even if we look at them from unusual angles and views. The important brain areas involved in these processes are the occipital and parietal lobes.

After head injury, individuals may have difficulty in recognizing a range of visual information, although this is not a particularly common consequence.

How are visual perception difficulties seen in everyday life?

Your relative may have difficulty in recognizing objects if they are not in their usual places or are placed at a funny angle (e.g. if their clothes are in a jumble or their reading glasses are put down in an unusual place). In contrast, if they are laid out clearly and in a familiar place, they can easily identify the same objects. As their eyes are working perfectly well, glasses will not help correct this type of problem.

Changes in visuospatial skills

These are the skills we use to make spatial judgements e.g. judging how near something or someone is, judging depths, constructing objects and putting things together (e.g. DIY projects), and finding our way around indoors and outside (e.g. following simple routes). Again, these processes involve the occipital and parietal lobes.

How are spatial difficulties seen in everyday life?

Difficulties with spatial skills may result in individuals over- (or under-) reaching for things, having problems judging the depth of steps and stairs, or being unable to judge how far away an approaching car is when crossing the road. These can be very frightening and confusing experiences. They may also become disoriented when they are out or when trying to find their way around a building, or when trying to follow a map. In addition, DIY tasks and other jobs that require visualizing where things need to go are much more difficult.

Other cognitive difficulties

Other cognitive difficulties less commonly seen after head injury include those mentioned below.

Agnosia/difficulties in recognition

This relates to difficulty in recognizing objects even though they can be seen perfectly well. In these cases, the individual has lost his/her ability to recognize and identify previously well-known objects. Visual agnosia can be confusing and disorientating, and may be difficult to spot initially.

Apraxia

This relates to problems in carrying out particular movements (e.g. cleaning teeth, getting dressed). Specific difficulties are experienced in thinking about and planning movements. Such difficulties may be caused by other problems (e.g. physical limitations) and these must be ruled out before diagnosing apraxia. As a result, the injured individual may find it hard to follow commands or complete tasks in a certain order. This may sometimes look like clumsiness.

Visual neglect

After a head injury, individuals can sometimes be unaware of one side of space (ignoring things on one side, or ignoring one side of their body). This is a form of attentional problem and is called neglect. Visual neglect is relatively unusual after head injury.

Coping with changes in thinking skills

In the early stages of recovery, family members are understandably most focused on medical and physical issues, and questions such as 'Will my relative ever regain consciousness?' and 'Will my relative pull through?' dominate. After this stage, relatives start to ask 'Will he/she ever walk or talk again?' Concerns about cognitive (thinking) changes tend to occur slightly later still. If such changes are subtle, families may only become aware of them after some time (perhaps after their relative returns to work). Even with more severe changes, the full impact of these difficulties is only really likely to be felt on return to the family home.

If your relative is experiencing some form of change in their thinking abilities, you might be very worried and confused about the nature of these changes, especially if you do not fully understand what is happening to your relative or if you have not received information on these problems. Depending on the nature and severity of the difficulties, you might have additional worries about leaving your relative alone for safety reasons, worry about them returning to work, or about how they are coping with everyday stressors. Dealing with this can be extremely tiring and frustrating.

Ways to help your relative with cognitive problems

As discussed in Chapter 2, we expect to see improvements over time as the brain spontaneously mends. During this process of natural recovery (which is most marked over the first year or two) improvements in cognitive functioning are likely. However, it is impossible to predict how much recovery there will be and when this will stop. It is realistic to say that, with more moderate and severe head injuries, persisting changes in some areas of cognition are likely.

Unfortunately, there is not a great deal that you or your relative can do to have a direct influence on the natural recovery of most of these thinking and memory functions. While there is some evidence that attention can be exercised or 'trained' to improve, you generally cannot speed up the process of recovery by regularly exercising and testing out other functions like memory. Research shows that this type of approach usually does not help much in reducing the impact of such difficulties in everyday life or cure these problems. If your relative has received specialist rehabilitation you may already be familiar with this idea. You may have been told that memory is not like a muscle that can be strengthened by repeatedly exercising it (e.g. by using memory games). If you have not had contact with rehabilitation professionals, this may be a surprising message to hear. You may find it upsetting or frustrating, as it can sound as if there is nothing you can do to help your relative. However, this is *not* the case.

> ❌ **Myth** Repeatedly exercising memory and other areas of cognition helps 'cure' problems by restoring functioning in those areas.
>
> ❗ **Fact** Cognitive processes, such as memory, improve spontaneously over time independently of what you do. It is more helpful to practise everyday tasks rather than more 'abstract' games.

What can help?

While it is certainly not worth you spending all your time encouraging your relative to 'exercise' their memory repeatedly, there are still many other useful things you can do which can improve the situation and help you all 'bypass' and cope with the changes. Even in the case of attention, where repetitive exercises may be recommended to improve functioning, this would just be one approach adopted. It is also important to look at other ways to reduce the impact of problems with attention in everyday life.

It is important to seek personalized information about your relative's head injury and understand the specific cognitive difficulties they are experiencing. This is because every head injury is unique and the difficulties experienced can be so varied. Rather than ask 'Does my relative have a memory problem?', ask 'What types of things is my relative finding difficult to remember?', 'How severe is the memory problem?', 'Is his/her memory for other things OK?', 'How will we be able to help him manage these memory problems?', and 'Who can advise us on this issue?'. Finding the answers to these questions can guide you towards the strategies that will be most effective in your relative's case.

Resources which provide more detailed information and advice for dealing with particular patterns of cognitive problems are listed at the end of this book. However, we provide some very general guidance below.

Whatever the type of cognitive change you have noticed, we know that the general recommendations outlined in Chapter 1 should be helpful. Making some basic changes to your relative's home and work environments (e.g. reducing distractions) and using a range of simple compensatory strategies and aids (such as diaries and lists, or a dossett box to aid taking medication) can have dramatic effects. A dossett box, for example, is a simple plastic box that has separate spaces for each day's medication. This can be filled up in advance and can reduce the likelihood of your relative forgetting to take or mixing up their daily medication (thus enhancing their control and independence in this area). In addition, providing more time to complete everyday tasks, planning ahead, and having a predictable routine to the week can all help to reduce pressure and tension within the family.

We noted earlier that some people have reservations about adopting these types of approaches. People often think that it is better for their relative to be 'pushed' to try things out without any help or clues—even if this means that they will make mistakes. For example, some people might think that it is better for their relative to guess where something is (thus testing their memory) rather than put up a label on a cupboard (which may feel like cheating or making things too easy for the person with memory problems). You often hear people say 'If you don't use it you'll lose it'. However, this is *not* accurate.

In the case of memory problems, we know that using memory aids (like a diary or a wall planner) and finding other ways of getting around memory difficulties is much more effective than trying to exercise memory by doing repetitive tasks and tests. We know that using memory aids is in no way detrimental and does not hinder any natural recovery of memory that may occur. On the whole, it is much better to use strategies and support individuals with memory problems in such a way that they do not have the opportunity to guess and make mistakes when they are trying to learn something or do something new. Why?

> We know that with more severe memory problems, learning is best achieved by **repetition and routine**. This is somewhat different to how people without memory problems learn. We are much more likely to learn through **trial and error** (i.e. learn through making mistakes). However, this only works for us because we can remember the mistakes we made next time we are in the same situation—and we can then do something different! In contrast, if you cannot remember your mistakes, being allowed to get things wrong can cause many additional problems (the mistake can actually get in the way of learning the right response).

Some of the self-help resources listed at the end of this book include information on practical strategies to address thinking and memory problems. It is important to look through these to get some ideas, and then try some out to see what works best for your relative and the family. If your relative has only mild difficulties, they may be able to use these resources themselves to develop their own strategies. If their problems are more severe, other family members may need to take a lead role in this.

In some cases (if the problems are complex, difficult to understand, or severe) a formal assessment by a specialist professional such as a clinical neuropsychologist may be useful. He/she will undertake tests that will help identify the exact nature of your relative's difficulties and advise you on the strategies that will be most helpful.

Ways to help yourself

It can be very frustrating and draining to support someone with significant cognitive problems. Family members often describe how their relative's cognitive changes have a major impact on everyone in the family. Resulting changes for family members frequently include having to be more vigilant about their relative's safety, taking an increased role in organizing and 'remembering' for that person (e.g. reminding them of things they need to do), and constantly trying to motivate or encourage their relative to do more. As described in Chapter 9, family roles and duties may also change significantly, especially if your relative has been unable to return to work or resume domestic duties such as managing finances or helping the children with their homework. Family members may also feel the effects of cognitive changes in other ways. For example, their relative may forget important birthdays and anniversaries, show a lack of interest in everyday events (such as children's school events/achievements), and display much higher levels of irritability than previously. Everyone (particularly children) may need to adapt their behaviour (e.g. being much quieter than before) in order to reduce the problems experienced. These changes in family life can be difficult to adjust to, effortful, and tiring.

It is important to understand fully what is happening in order to prevent family members misinterpreting or 'taking personally' issues arising out of cognitive problems. Remember that, although extremely frustrating, memory lapses and other problems caused by changes in thinking abilities are not deliberate—making mistakes and forgetfulness are symptoms of the head injury.

It can be helpful to talk to wider family and friends about the cognitive problems your relative is experiencing so that they also understand and can provide support. It may also ensure that they do not place unnecessary demands and stresses on your relative, which can have a knock-on effect on you and the rest of the family.

 Frequently asked questions

 ◆ **Will my relative's memory ever improve?**

After a head injury we expect to see some changes over time as the brain spontaneously mends. During this process of natural recovery (especially over the first year or two) improvements in all areas, including cognition, are likely. We know that cognitive problems tend to recover more slowly than physical problems. However, it is impossible to predict how much recovery there will be after a head injury and when this will stop. It is realistic to say that with more moderate and severe head injuries long-term enduring change in some areas is highly likely, and 100% recovery is highly unlikely. However, this message about recovery is not as bleak as it sounds. Often families report changes for many years after the head injury as people continue to adjust to and find ways around their difficulties. Even when spontaneous recovery slows down or stops, there are ways of managing cognitive problems so that everyday functioning continues to improve.

 ◆ **Will my relative remember what has happened to him/her?**

This is a question that can cause family members much worry, especially if their loved one sustained their head injury in very traumatic circumstances. Although older memories are usually well preserved, it is unusual for people to remember the events leading up to the head injury itself. This period of memory loss, referred to as retrograde amnesia, differs in length between individuals and can be hours, days, or months before the injury occurred. In all cases, memory for the accident itself is never retrieved.

◆ **Why do my relative's difficulties seem to vary over time?**

Cognitive difficulties may become much more evident when your relative is tired or is feeling physically unwell. From your own experiences, you will know that it is harder to concentrate or learn new information when you are tired or unwell, even if you do not normally have problems in these areas. This effect is magnified after a head injury. In addition, factors in the home and work environment may exaggerate the difficulties—for example, if the office is very noisy or there are lots of people visiting at home, your relative may find it harder to cope with tasks that he/she is usually able to do without too much difficulty.

◆ **I've been told that exercising memory doesn't help, but shouldn't I be encouraging my relative to keep their mind stimulated?**

It certainly won't do any harm to encourage your relative to engage in activities that they enjoy and find stimulating (e.g. puzzles, reading). Just be aware that putting a lot of effort into memory games and activities is unlikely to result in changes that can be seen in everyday life.

◆ **How will we know if strategies are working?**

Signs that strategies are effective might include finding that your relative is experiencing more success in everyday tasks, that you are having to prompt them less, that they are showing fewer signs of frustration and distress, or that stress levels within the family are not so high.

◆ **'My relative doesn't seem to be aware of the problems he has with concentrating and remembering. How can I help him understand that he can't do some of the things he used to do easily?**

This is a particularly hard area for family members to address. We know that after head injury individuals sometimes show no or only limited awareness of the changes experienced. They may not fully appreciate what has happened to them and what their current abilities are—thus they may place themselves in risky situations. Families are often trying to get the balance right between being encouraging (and maintaining their relative's independence), and giving their relative realistic feedback about their difficulties and keeping them out of danger. If your relative has poor awareness of their difficulties, they may get angry and upset, and may see you as being overly critical. Giving them feedback on areas of difficulty is best done slowly and sensitively, with support or back-up from professionals. Information and feedback from health care professionals who know your relative well (if they are receiving rehabilitation) can be useful and may redirect anger and frustration away from you or other family members.

6

Changes in speech, language, and communication

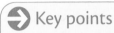 **Key points**

- Difficulties with communication can result from damage to the parts of the brain responsible for speech and language.

- The severity and type of disorder seen will depend on the location and extent of damage.

- There are several types of communication disorder, affecting different aspects of speech and language. A combination of these can occur after head injury.

- Speech, language, and communication difficulties can have a major impact on everyday life, and can cause frustration and distress for family members.

- A speech and language therapist (SALT) can help assess the nature of communication disorder and help you understand how to facilitate communication with your relative.

Common speech, language, and communication difficulties after head injury: an overview

There are several different types of communication disorder that can result from damage to the brain. The type and severity of these problems will depend on:

- the location and extent of the brain injury

- the severity of the damage

- the stage of recovery.

In most people the key areas of the brain responsible for controlling speech and language are located in the left hemisphere (side) of the brain. However, the right hemisphere controls other communication skills, and control of the muscles of speech depends on several different areas of the brain.

The types of communication disorder that can occur following a head injury are:

- **aphasia** (sometimes called dysphasia)
- **verbal dyspraxia**
- **dysarthria**.

It is quite common in head injury to see a combination of these disorders, especially in the early stages of recovery. This is because head injury affects diffuse areas of the brain, rather than a precise location as may be seen following a stroke.

Aphasia

Aphasia is a speech and language disorder which can affect all aspects of language:

- understanding what is said to you
- the ability to find words and sounds to speak
- the ability to read and write.

There is a wide range of severity and types of aphasia and each individual will present slightly differently. It can be very frustrating for a person who is aphasic (and their relatives) as the person is often fully aware of what they want to say and their intelligence is intact, but their ability to communicate is impaired. A person with aphasia described it as feeling as though 'their computer was working fine but the connection to the printer was broken'.

The effects that aphasia might have on your relative are shown in Table 6.1.

Verbal dyspraxia

Verbal **dyspraxia** is the name given to another speech problem that is usually seen alongside aphasia to some degree. It relates to a difficulty in programming and sequencing the movements of the speech muscles to make speech sounds and sequence those sounds in words. In mild dyspraxia there may just be mild sound errors in words or difficulty in saying long complex words. In severe dyspraxia (sometimes called apraxia) the person is unable to make any deliberate speech sounds at all.

Dysarthria

Dysarthria is a speech difficulty caused by weakness or difficulty in moving and coordinating the muscles used for speaking. These include the respiratory muscles (muscles for breath control), larynx (voice box), soft palate, tongue, and lips. These muscles produce voice and speech sounds in rapidly coordinated

Table 6.1 Effects of aphasia

	Mild to moderate difficulties	Severe difficulties
Understanding Things that are heard or read (receptive difficulties)	Person is able to follow short spoken phrases but has difficulty following long complex instructions or information spoken to him/her	Person has difficulty understanding anything that is said to him/her, even single words
Reading Ability to read may be preserved in some individuals after a head injury but their ability to understand and make sense of what they are reading can be impaired; this can cause them some confusion	Able to read single words or short phrases (e.g. newspaper headlines), but unable to read, process, and retain long paragraphs	Unable to read single words and understand them
Speaking Expressive difficulties	Occasional to frequent difficulties in finding the correct word that the person wants to say; occasional to frequent use of incorrect words or mispronunciation of words causing speech to be less fluent. A person may have additional verbal dyspraxia. The person may be able to speak occasional single words or short phrases only, or they may be able to speak fluently but the majority of the words do not make sense	Unable to express themselves verbally at all
Writing This can be affected by aphasia, which may be in addition to any difficulty the person might have in controlling the hand for writing.	May be able to write words and sentences but makes occasional spelling errors	Unable to spell or write single words; in less severe cases may be able to write or point to the first letter of a word on an alphabet chart

movements when we speak. In pure dysarthria a person's language (ability to find words and sequence them into a sentence) is intact but their ability to speak is impaired at the levels of breath control and/or of voice and speech production.

◆ **Mild dysarthria** A person is able to speak in long sentences but their speech sounds slightly slurred as their articulation is affected. Their voice may be slightly altered (e.g. slightly gruff, quiet, nasal, or over-loud) or their intonation and prosody (e.g. the rhythm, stress placement in words and sentences, and variations in tone and expression in the voice) may be affected—for example, they may sound monotone and flat or their speech may have a jerky rhythm.

◆ **Severe dysarthria** In its most severe form a person is unable to move their speech muscles voluntarily at all and therefore is unable to speak (this is called anarthria). This is often accompanied by severe eating and swallowing difficulties (see Chapter 4). In a slightly less severe case a person may be able to make occasional speech sounds or single words.

The impact of cognitive problems on communication

The cognitive difficulties typically associated with head injury (such as problems with memory, organization, planning and sequencing, drawing inference, and reasoning) can all have a significant impact on a person's communication skills. For example, they can affect conversation skills such as being able to listen, take turns, and retain and process (make sense of) what someone has said, and the ability to plan and sequence their response. These difficulties may be very obvious or subtle.

People in low awareness state

It may be that your relative has sustained a very severe brain injury and remains in an apparently uncommunicative state (different levels of awareness and responsiveness after head injury such as coma, low awareness states, and vegetative conditions are described in Chapter 2). Having a relative with this type of difficulty raises obvious concerns about communication. Families are frequently concerned about how best to communicate with their relative, how to establish what their relative understands and is aware of, and how communication can be improved. Some families can feel very despondent and disheartened about communicating with an apparently unresponsive relative and may 'give up' talking to them if they remain in this state for some time. This is an extremely stressful time for all involved as it is often very difficult to know for sure how much a person who is in a low state of awareness can hear and understand.

It is not uncommon for families to feel as if the hospital staff are 'missing' the injured person's efforts to communicate, or that the staff do not believe their reports of their relative's attempts to communicate. It can be a time of conflict and upset, but it is important to try to work together to gain a broad picture of the injured person's communication abilities. There are several useful assessment tools (based on very close and frequent observation of the injured person) that can help to monitor changes in a person's level of awareness and ability to communicate. Head injury rehabilitation staff can advise you further about these.

Ways to help your relative with communication difficulties:

People who experience speech and language difficulties often describe them as one of the most frustrating and upsetting problems following a head injury. Communication difficulties can cause a great deal of frustration, distress, and upset in family relationships. You might find, for example, that others in the family automatically speak for the person with the communication difficulty, bypass them in conversation, or constantly correct their speech. Family members might lack the patience to deal with the communication difficulties, or be reluctant to accept and use other means of communication. The individual with the communication difficulties may also express more feelings of frustration when experiencing problems communicating with others—and may become more withdrawn or reliant on other family members as a result.

In the acute stages following head injury a person who is experiencing communication difficulties should be referred to a speech and language therapist (SALT). Your GP should be able to organize this. A SALT is able to assess the nature and severity of communication difficulties and provide advice and guidance on how to help the person communicate. During the rehabilitation stages there are a wide range of speech and language therapy approaches and strategies which may aid recovery and help the person communicate, depending on the nature and severity of the difficulty. Talk to staff about the strategies that will be most helpful for your relative.

A general principle is to think of communication as more than just speech. Gesture, facial expression, writing, eye movements, looking at or pointing to written words, or drawing pictures can all be very communicative. Encourage and accept all means of communication open to someone (often called **total communication**), and do not be afraid to use them yourself. Initially it can feel 'silly' or embarrassing to be using lots of gestures or drawing information that you want to communicate, but once you have got used to using these strategies your relative is likely to gain a lot of benefit from them.

If your relative has **difficulty in understanding** what others say, try the following.

- Use short phrases, one at a time.
- Support what you say by writing down key words.

- Use natural gestures to support your speech (this may be easier to understand).

- Use pictures of the key topic or item to support your speech (to support understanding of the words).

- Reduce background noise and distraction (e.g. turn off the radio when talking, and avoid several people talking at once).

- Signal a change in topic of conversation clearly.

- Provide key information written down in short phrases, and highlight key words.

If your relative has **difficulty expressing him/herself**, try the following.

- Allow time.

- It may help to ask closed questions, i.e. questions that can be answered with 'yes' or 'no'.

- The person with expressive difficulties may be able to write or spell out the first letter or whole words on an alphabet chart.

- Write down options for your relative to point to (to assist in choice-making). Help your relative to answer open questions by providing written single word/short phrase options to select from (e.g. for the question 'What did you do at the weekend?', write out options such as 'stayed at home', 'went for a drive', 'trip out', 'visitors').

- Similarly, use pictures to help communication.

- A communication chart or book of key words or pictures to communicate everyday needs or about the person's family, likes and dislikes, interests, area they live, etc. may assist communication. A SALT can advise on compiling this.

- Encourage all means of communication, e.g. the use of gesture, writing, or drawing to support speech.

- Keep a pen and paper to hand to enable easy use by someone in conversation with someone with speech difficulties.

Use of some of the strategies outlined above (adapted to your relative's particular pattern of difficulties) can help reduce some of the feelings of frustration and distress you may all be experiencing.

Specialist communication devices

The general strategies listed above include what we call low-tech communication aids. These are simple aids to communication (such as communication books, picture or word charts) and props that you can develop to act as 'ramps' to assist in communication, much like a ramp up a step assists mobility. These can include pictures, photos, and maps that centre around a topic of conversation.

There is also a wide range of higher-tech (electronic) communication aids, which are sometimes recommended after specialist assessment by a SALT.

One example of such a specialist communication device is a **lightwriter.** This is a small text-based aid with a screen that displays a typed message to the person to whom the injured person is 'talking'. Other examples include computer-based systems accessed via a switch. These switches can be adapted to overcome physical problems (such as problems with moving a hand) so that the switch is operated by a head movement (if the injured person is able to this).

Coping with a relative in an uncommunicative state

As outlined earlier, a small number of people with severe head injury may not recover their ability to communicate and may appear to remain in a minimally aware and uncommunicative state. This can be distressing for families to understand and cope with. Staff working with your relative can advise on particular strategies that might be helpful but in general the following can be useful.

♦ Continue to talk normally to your relative, although we acknowledge that it can be very difficult to maintain this over time, especially if the person does not appear to be making further recovery. It is especially important to try to keep your relative informed about what is going on and what their treatment involves. Many families wonder whether it is helpful to give the injured person detailed information about what has happened to them. It is difficult to give general advice on this issue and should be considered on an individual basis. Generally it is probably adequate to tell them that they have had an accident, that they are in hospital and being looked after, and that family are present.

♦ Try your best to keep all communication clear, simple, and relevant to their interests and preferences (e.g. share news about family members, give them updates on how their favourite football team is doing). Use 'total communication' principles by bringing in taped recordings of family messages, favourite music, and photographs.

♦ Try to avoid 'non-specific' ways of communicating such as noisy 'toys' or flashing lights. It can be tempting to think that these might 'stimulate' your relative into communicating again, but they are more likely to tire and confuse them, making communication more unlikely. It is also helpful to avoid trying to stimulate your relative with toys and games that are not appropriate for their age. Encourage other family members to do the same.

♦ Try to be patient and work towards small improvements over time. Head-injured people do not generally wake up from coma in the way portrayed in Hollywood films.

♦ Make sure that you have support for yourself and your family.

Ways to help yourself

Problems with communication can be extremely frustrating and upsetting for the whole family, as well as for the individual with these difficulties. As the people closest to the injured individual, and perhaps spending most time with them on a daily basis, family members are most likely to be affected by problems with communication. For example, you might find it draining to think constantly about what and how you communicate with your relative or having to work much harder to establish what they are trying to say to you, especially as talking to each other is something we very much take for granted. You might also find it upsetting if you see your relative becoming frustrated, isolated, or less confident as a result of their communication difficulties.

Hopefully, the types of approaches outlined above will help you and your relative to reduce frustration and maximize your relative's ability to communicate with you. It can also be very helpful to talk to others (e.g. friends and the wider family) about the communication problems your relative is experiencing so that they also understand and can provide some support. Sharing strategies and ways to support and facilitate communication with your relative may help both parties enjoy their interactions more, reduce frustration, and help maintain their old relationships.

Taking time out for yourself can also give both you and your relative a break from each other and make your time together more positive.

Get specialist support from others if you feel that you do not fully understand what the difficulties are or you feel that you are not managing them well. You can approach your GP or head injury service (if one exists in your area), or contact one of the support organizations suggested at the end of this book. Remember that a SALT can provide specialist advice that is tailored to your relative's individual needs.

 Frequently asked questions

◆ **Will my relative's speech ever improve?**

Recovery and improvement of speech and language disorders depends, like other problems after head injury, on a number of factors, and differs for each person. Factors affecting improvement include:

- ◆ the type of speech problem
- ◆ the severity of the disorder
- ◆ the ability of the person to engage in and respond to therapy
- ◆ the presence of other difficulties that may affect recovery e.g. cognitive difficulties or medical complications
- ◆ support and communication opportunities.

Although your relative's ability to communicate may improve with time, it is important to find ways around any ongoing difficulties using compensatory strategies and techniques such as those discussed in this chapter.

You might find, that after head injury you have to communicate in a different way with your relative. Use of pictures or writing to aid communication is not going to hinder recovery in any way and these may provide valuable ways of maximizing your relative's ability to express him/herself and reduce any feelings of frustration.

Will it help to practice writing the alphabet?

This depends on the nature of the speech problem. Writing practice may help some people, but for others this can add to frustration and gain nothing. Seeking specific advice from a speech and language therapist (SALT) is advised if you are unsure about this.

Will it help to read to the person?

If you are able to ask the person with the communication problem whether they would like this, then please ask. Some people who enjoy reading the paper or a magazine, but now struggle to do so, may find this enjoyable, especially if you are able to have some form of discussion about an article afterwards. Keep communicating.

Will it help to raise my voice?

No, unless there is a hearing problem. People with speech problems often report that other people speak to them loudly or treat them as if they are 'stupid' and this is very insulting. Speak to your relative in a normal calm voice, and if the person has problems with understanding, it may help to ask one question or give one piece of information at a time.

Where can I get more speech and language therapy?

If you feel that you and your relative need specialist assessment and advice from a SALT, contact one of the organizations mentioned earlier (details are provided at the end of this book) or ask your GP or head injury service to find out what services exists in your area and how to access these. Community speech and language therapy services tend to be stretched thinly, so you may not get as much input as you would like. Sometimes, however, it is not more speech and language therapy that is needed but help with coming to terms with living with a communication disability (along with other acquired disabilities). The charity UKConnect can provide excellent information, publications, and courses (see www. ukconnect.org). Again, details are at the end of the book. Support from counselling and psychology services may also be helpful.

7

Changes in emotions and behaviour

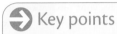 Key points

◆ Changes in behaviour and emotions often occur after a head injury.

◆ The causes of such changes are often 'invisible' to others and not easily understood.

◆ They are typically the most upsetting consequences of head injury for relatives and are associated with poorer long-term outcomes.

◆ The changes seen relate to the areas of brain damaged. They also arise for other reasons (e.g. reactions to the consequences of the head injury).

◆ Although these problems are challenging and stressful, their impact can be minimized by making some changes to the environment and altering the demands placed on the person with a head injury.

If you feel that you are unable to cope with these changes, or feel in any way unsafe, seek support from professional services via your GP.

Common emotional and behavioural changes after head injury: an overview

A head injury often has a significant effect on a person's emotions and behaviour. After head injury, changes in emotional responses to situations, and the ability to control emotions and behaviour can all occur. These difficulties have been shown to be the hardest for families to cope with.

Common emotional reactions after brain injury include:

◆ **depression**

◆ **anxiety and fear**

◆ **anger**

◆ **frustration**

◆ **mood swings** and feeling less in control of emotions than previously.

Common behaviour changes include:

- **apathy** or **reduced motivation**
- **increased irritability**
- **aggressive behaviour** (physical or verbal)
- **socially inappropriate** behaviour (e.g. swearing, saying hurtful things to people)
- **trouble relating to others**
- **restlessness/agitation**.

The actual changes seen, and their severity, depend on a range of factors including the severity of the head injury, the areas of brain damaged, your relative's situation (e.g. how able they are to return to work and home duties), how your relative copes with stress, and the type of person they were before the head injury.

You may notice that your relative's reactions to situations has changed (e.g. they may be less tolerant of others and be much more irritable than previously), or they may be reacting to situations in a similar but much more pronounced way. Many people feel as though their relative's personality has changed.

Like the cognitive changes described previously, these emotional and behavioural changes are often difficult to understand and cause high levels of distress for all concerned. These changes may not be obvious initially, or may be put down to other reasons (e.g. the stress of being in hospital). Your relative may have come home without anyone talking to you about these issues. In addition, the causes of emotional and behavioural changes are 'hidden' (especially if the person has no physical problems) and thus are hard for others to understand and know how best to provide you with support. Therefore these changes may be overlooked or misinterpreted by others. It can be very difficult and exhausting to live with someone whose behaviour is unpredictable and difficult to manage, or who is showing high levels of emotional distress. Often these feelings and behaviours are directed at you and other family members, as the people closest to them.

Why do emotional and behaviour changes occur?

A variety of factors contribute to the changes described above (Figure 7.1).

The direct effects of the head injury

First we have the direct (or primary) effects of the head injury itself. Damage to the areas of the brain that regulate our emotions and behaviour (particularly the limbic system and the frontal lobes) can result in significant changes. Chemical imbalances within the brain, which may directly influence mood, can also arise after head injury.

Unfortunately, the brain areas most involved in controlling behaviour, the frontal lobes, are also the most vulnerable to damage. They are particularly important

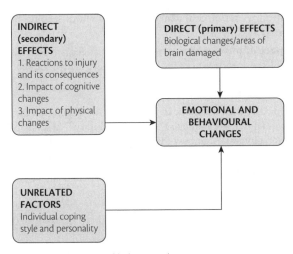

Figure 7.1 Causes of emotional and behaviour changes

in the moderation of behaviour, i.e. playing a role in inhibiting (stopping) our responses (e.g. saying something that would be embarrassing or upsetting to others) and being aware of ourselves and our behaviour (insight) and its impact on other people.

The indirect effects of the head injury

There are also secondary or indirect effects of the head injury. These include the following.

◆ **The psychological reactions to the injury and its consequences** It is important to remember that your relative has experienced a sudden traumatic event. As a result they may be coping with a great deal of uncertainty, may feel out of control, and may be unable to do things that they used to do. Thus it is understandable that they may be experiencing a whole array of emotions, including low mood, anger, anxiety, and frustration, as well as reduced confidence and loss of self-esteem.

◆ **The impact of cognitive changes** Cognitive problems can also contribute to emotional and behavioural changes. If the injured individual has slowed thinking speed, impaired attention, or memory difficulties, they may find that they have fewer thinking resources to work through problems and deal with stresses. This will make them more prone to irritability or displaying angry outbursts. Feeling confused, disoriented, or being unable to remember things can also give rise to feelings of distress. In addition, cognitive changes can result in a loss of confidence in one's abilities leading to emotional problems.

◆ **The impact of physical factors** Physical changes, which include fatigue, sleep problems, incontinence, and pain, may have a large influence on mood.

Unrelated factors

Finally, the picture seen after a head injury will also depend on factors specific to that individual that are unrelated to the head injury. These include the individual's personality traits and how they usually cope with stress. Some of us are more prone than others to emotional disorders such as anxiety and depression.

It can be very difficult to identify one particular cause for the changes seen and often a combination of factors is responsible.

Emotional disorders

Depression

Depression is a common emotional response after head injury. We know from research and clinical experience that the rate of depression is significantly greater among people with head injury than among the general population. It is estimated that approximately half of people experience depression at some stage after a head injury. Although it can occur at any stage, it is more common in the later stages of recovery (as recovery rate starts to slow down or plateau). In fact, your relative may be protected from depression in the early stages of their recovery if they have reduced insight (see Chapter 5). They may become more prone to depression as insight improves and they realize the long-term nature of their difficulties, or when they are faced with their difficulties on an everyday basis.

Someone who has had a head injury may become depressed for a variety of reasons. These fall into the broad categories outlined earlier. Depression may be due to direct changes to the brain (e.g. disruption in the brain chemistry) or indirect psychological factors (e.g. the possible loss of their job, their roles within family, future plans, loss of friendships, and loss of themselves as they were before).

The term depression is sometimes used inaccurately. It is important to be aware that depression is different from short episodes of feeling low, and requires different action. Fluctuations in mood and periods of feeling low and tearful are common reactions after head injury, and can occur without your relative actually being 'clinically' depressed. Depression is much more severe—it endures over time (at least 2 weeks) and prevents the individual getting on with day-to-day life. Symptoms of depression include:

◆ feelings of great sadness

◆ feelings of hopelessness about the future

- reduced ability to concentrate
- loss of interest and motivation
- changes in appetite
- problems sleeping
- suicidal thoughts and feelings.

It can sometimes be difficult to diagnose depression after a head injury, as many symptoms, such as poor concentration and irritability, are the same for both head injury and depression. Professional support and advice—from your relative's GP in the first instance—may be necessary in order to assess this properly.

If your relative also has difficulties in speaking and communicating how they are feeling, it can be particularly difficult to ascertain whether they are depressed. If you are concerned that they are showing some signs of being depressed, raise this issue with their doctor or other health professionals involved in their care. Support from a speech and language therapist (SALT) may be necessary in such cases.

Anger and irritability

Some people describe living with their relative after injury as being like 'walking on eggshells' in order to prevent angry outbursts. Again, there are many potential reasons for this change. Anger problems may arise directly from the brain damage itself; damage to the frontal lobes can result in poor anger control. In contrast, your relative may be expressing feelings of anger and frustration in reaction to their circumstances and the things that they cannot do. Outbursts may also reflect cognitive changes and reduced resources for coping successfully with everyday frustrations. Such difficulties may be more apparent when your relative is tired or overwhelmed.

Emotional lability

Emotionalism (or emotional lability) is when someone is unable to control their emotions. This is due to the direct effects of the brain damage. Individuals may find that they burst into tears or laughter more easily than previously, which may be triggered by events that would normally make people laugh or feel sad, or may come 'out of the blue'. Whatever the trigger, the individual may feel that their response is out of control or out of proportion to the situation, which can cause them embarrassment. It is an effect of brain injury that is not easily understood by others.

If your relative is having specific difficulty with emotional lability, you and your relative (and the rest of the family) may need to sit down and agree ways of handling this. Medication can sometimes help control emotional outbursts. If emotional lability is a major issue for your relative it may be worth discussing this with their GP or another doctor involved in their care.

Anxiety and fear

Feeling worried and scared is perfectly understandable when you consider the changes that the injured person is experiencing. Anxiety and fear can take many forms and are relatively common responses to head injury. Your relative may feel more anxious generally, or they may develop more specific worries. Such specific worries may be about their health (e.g. having an epileptic seizure), the future (e.g. returning to work), social situations (e.g. meeting old friends), and changes in physical abilities (e.g. fear of falling). Your relative may develop a phobia (extreme anxiety) about particular situations or objects and experience symptoms of panic, and thus avoid these situations whenever possible. If your relative was an anxious person before their injury, or had specific worries, these may become worse. As a result, individuals may become less confident and more dependent on other family members. They may try to avoid doing certain things for themselves (asking you or other family members instead) or not want to be alone.

Post-traumatic stress disorder (PTSD)

PTSD is an extreme form of anxiety disorder which can also occur after head injury. It typically develops after an individual has been involved in or witnesses a life-threatening traumatic event that is outside normal experience. Symptoms include emotional numbness, avoidance of reminders of the event, nightmares and 'flashbacks' (which occur frequently and uncontrollably), and feeling constantly 'on edge' and on the look out for danger. We now know that people can experience symptoms of PTSD after a head injury even if it is severe and they cannot remember the details of the traumatic event itself. The precise numbers of people who develop PTSD after head injury are unavailable; however we do know that this is a relatively rare reaction. If you have concerns that your relative is showing signs of PTSD please discuss this with your GP or another health care professional in the first instance. They can refer you on for expert advice and support.

Emotional numbness

Individuals can also show a 'blunting' in their emotional responses. They may show no emotion and fail to show any response to events or people who previously would have elicited an emotional reaction (e.g. if their children are upset or hurt). Again, this can be a direct effect of the head injury (specifically damage to the front and top of the frontal lobes), or arise from other reasons (e.g. mood disorders such as depression or PTSD). Although very different from the emotional disorders described above, this lack of emotion can be as distressing for others in the family as for the relative themselves.

Behaviour changes

Behaviour changes occurring after head injury usually cause high levels of distress for families. Family members may feel that their injured relative is 'not the same person that they were before'. In addition, the underlying cause of the behaviour is normally invisible to others, and so families often do not get a sympathetic response when their relative behaves oddly. Behaviour changes may cause distress for the individual with the head injury if they are aware of them. More frequently however, individuals are unaware that their behaviour has changed, or is upsetting or offensive to others. We have already discussed one aspect of behaviour change—increased irritability and angry outbursts. Other typical behaviour changes include becoming:

- impulsive
- disinhibited
- egocentric (self-centred)
- passive and withdrawn.

Impulsive behaviour

The direct effects of injuries to the frontal lobes may result in impulsive behaviour. If your relative is impulsive, they will react quickly to situations without thinking through the issues and options, and may place him/herself in potentially risky situations as a result (e.g. moving quickly out of a wheelchair without putting the brakes on, making an impulsive decision, speaking impulsively).

Disinhibition

Individuals may become disinhibited in their behaviour (again, this is directly related to frontal lobe injuries). Disinhibition means that the individual says or does things that other people would not do in the same situation and that they would not have done before their injury. They may become very outspoken, losing their social graces, swearing, or saying what they think about someone (even if this is upsetting, rude, or crude). It is as though the social 'brakes' we all normally use to stop ourselves saying or doing upsetting things no longer work well and behaviour goes 'unchecked'. They may also be self-neglectful (e.g. not being bothered with their appearance).

Egocentric behaviour

Individuals may become extremely focused on themselves and their own needs, and show little or no awareness of others' feelings. They may behave in ways that seem very selfish or childish to others. Usually this is a direct effect of damage to the frontal lobes and subsequent difficulties in thinking flexibly and being able to consider others' perspectives. This can be very upsetting to other family members, especially children, particularly if previously the individual was very caring and considerate to others.

Passivity and withdrawal

Some individuals become quite withdrawn and passive after a head injury, show no emotional responses, lose motivation, and find themselves unable to initiate (or get started on) any actions. Therefore they may not engage in activities they used to enjoy, or show little interest in things or people around them. As a result, individuals may appear lazy or deliberately awkward when they will not do anything without considerable nagging. It is important to remember that this is not the case. Although such problems usually reflect underlying frontal lobe damage, they may also be a symptom of depression. Input from a professional such as a doctor or clinical neuropsychologist may help tease these different factors out and establish the underlying cause of these difficulties.

> If your relative is showing aggressive or inappropriate behaviour, remember that this aspect of head injury is often the most difficult one for families to deal with. If your relative behaves in inappropriate ways, it is important for everyone to recognize that what they are seeing are the effects of head injury. Try not to take this behaviour personally or respond in an emotional manner (the latter can actually make the behaviour worse!). Instead, try to respond calmly and neutrally, and give clear feedback that the behaviour is inappropriate or makes you feel uncomfortable.

The impact of emotional problems on cognition

In the previous sections we have talked about cognition and emotions as quite separate entities. However, this is not the case, and it is important to consider how thinking and memory processes can also be affected by our emotions. If individuals are anxious about their memory or other areas of thinking, or are low in mood, they are likely to have greater difficulty in remembering, concentrating, and so on. From your own experience, you might be aware that when you are stressed or feeling low, you are more likely to be forgetful and unable to concentrate on tasks. This is a common response. For individuals who have cognitive problems, worrying is likely to exaggerate the existing cognitive problems. This may make them worry more or feel worse, and a vicious circle can quickly develop.

Other factors that may also impact on both cognition and mood include pain, tiredness, medication, and sleep problems. Speech difficulties (which may also occur after a head injury) can further complicate this picture. If someone is unable to talk about how they are feeling, emotional distress can be intensified.

Coping with emotional and behaviour changes

We know that the emotional and behavioural changes outlined above are usually the most distressing aspects of head injury for relatives to deal with. As we have already stated, it is often much easier to cope with physical changes (and to an extent, cognitive changes) if you feel that your loved one is still the same person as he/she was before their injury. As the head injury itself may be invisible to others (if your relative has made a good physical recovery), such changes are hard for other people to understand and thus support you with.

This means that families may not get a sympathetic response from others when their relative is behaving strangely or becomes very distressed. Sometimes people who did not know the person well before the injury occurred may overlook such changes. They may just view them as 'odd' or 'irritable', and as a result they may avoid contact with them. Therefore there is a danger that individuals, and their families, will become isolated. Children in particular may be very affected and embarrassed by these problems.

Ways to help your relative with emotional and behavioural problems

Collecting detailed and personalized information (e.g. about the times your relative shows difficult behaviours or expresses emotional distress) can help identify situations that trigger these feelings or behaviours.

Resources and self-help guides which provide specific advice on emotional and behavioural problems after head injury are also available (see Appendix 1). In addition, ideas from resources which advise on managing other areas of difficulty (e.g. problems in speaking or with memory) can help reduce everyday stresses and levels of emotional distress (for both your relative and yourself). Often small changes in the environment (such as reducing background noise or avoiding having too many visitors) and supporting your relative with their other problems can help reduce feelings of frustration and irritability. It may be possible to address some of these other areas of difficulty (e.g. with memory) fairly easily and in practical ways.

> If your relative is low in their mood, anxious, or showing other signs of emotional distress, remind them that their feelings (although frightening or upsetting at times) are perfectly natural. Listen to their worries and provide support, but look out for things that you do which might contribute to additional problems in the longer term.

It is important to seek professional input if the behaviour becomes too much for you or other family members to deal with. Talking therapies, such as counselling for your relative, or behavioural approaches (looking at different ways of managing difficult behaviour) can be helpful. Medication may also be used in some cases. You can talk to your relative's doctor about these options.

If you are very worried about your relative's emotional state

♦ Talk to your relative, offer to support them on a GP visit. Seek immediate professional support if you fear that your relative is experiencing high levels of emotional distress, such as depression or severe anxiety, or if they talk of suicide or harming themselves in any way and they do not feel able to seek help themselves. Their GP can advise on medication to help with this and also on other treatments available.

◆ Psychological approaches (talking therapies such as counselling, or more structured approaches like cognitive-behavioural therapy and behavioural therapy) can help your relative think about things differently, develop new coping strategies and skills, and influence behaviour. Usually a combination of antidepressant medication and psychological therapy is most effective. You can find out more about these by talking to the GP or other health professionals involved in your relative's care. If your relative wishes to access psychological support, their GP can refer them on to an NHS counsellor or clinical psychologist. Alternatively, you could access this privately. Ideally, you are looking for a therapist who specializes in head injury. You can ask the GP about this or you can contact one of the organizations listed in Appendix 1.

Ways to help yourself

As the people closest to the injured individual, family members are most likely to see and feel the effects of behaviour and emotional problems. Sometimes the injured person can behave more appropriately or show less distress when in other environments (e.g. with professionals within a rehabilitation unit). It is important not to take this too personally. This often happens because you are closest to your relative and thus the safest person to lash out at.

It is important to recognize that dealing with these types of difficult behaviours or emotional problems are extremely emotionally draining and there may be times when you feel unable to deal with them. See if you can recognize the times when you are less able to cope and feel as if you are running out of patience. Are there any early warning signs that things are getting too much for you? If possible have a break and take some time away.

Pay attention to how you are thinking about the problems you are seeing. Comparing your relative's behaviour before and after the head injury will tend to focus you on the negative changes, which will increase your distress. Instead, try to pay attention to positive aspects of your relative's behaviour and work towards not expecting it to be the same as it was before the injury.

If at any time you, or others in the family, feel unsafe, get away from the situation (e.g. leave the room if you feel the situation is getting out of control). Get support from others if you feel that you cannot cope with what is happening. You can approach your GP or contact one of the organizations listed in Appendix 1. Specialist professionals, such as a clinical psychologist, can provide advice on managing difficult behaviours.

In addition, access support for yourself and other family members as needed (whether this is informal support from friends and family or more professional support) if you feel that you are not coping well or feel very low or anxious yourself. Make sure that you take time to look after yourself—to rest and look after your own health needs. You might want to think about seeking counselling yourself. This may give you the time and opportunity to express your feelings about what has happened (e.g. grief, sadness at the changes in your relative). Do not underestimate the impact of your relative's behavioural and emotional changes on you and others.

❓ Frequently asked questions

* **Why does my relative seem more irritable and aggressive when they're at home with the family? Friends and rehab staff always seem to see them at their best**

The people closest to us are often the ones we feel safest 'hitting out' at. Therefore family members are most likely to see and feel the effects of behaviour and emotional problems after a head injury. It is important not to take this too personally.

* **Can I expect my relative's behaviour and/or mood to improve over time?**

Improvements over time are expected in the majority of cases. Sometimes the injured individual's control over emotions and behaviour increases as they recover. You might see improvements over time as those factors contributing to these problems (such as poor memory and concentration) also improve. Unfortunately, in some cases (particularly with more severe head injuries) the changes may be more enduring. However, there are many ways of managing these and reducing their impact on everyday life. Specialist input can help in some cases.

* **What should I do if I'm very worried about my relative's mood?**

If your relative appears very depressed or distressed, it is important to get specialist help as soon as possible. If possible, try to talk to your relative about this; offer to support them at a GP visit. If this is not possible, you should talk to their doctor in the first instance for advice.

8

Changes in sexual functioning

 Key points

- Changes in sexual functioning after head injury are common.

- Sexual activity is complex, involving physical, psychological, emotional, and social factors, and head injury may adversely affect all these.

- The impact of head injury on a relationship can be great and diverse, and the changes are experienced by the injured person and their partner.

- Help including specialist counselling, medication, and aids is available for sexual problems.

- Unresolved issues in the pre-existing relationship will tend to surface after head injury and may need to be talked about and managed.

Changes in sexual functioning: an overview

Sexual activity is complex. It involves physical, psychological, emotional, and social factors and head injury can affect it at each of these levels.

Sexual problems are common in the general population with one in 10 men reporting erectile problems. In a recent UK national survey, 15 per cent of women reported at least one 'persistent' sexual problem. In both sexes problems become more common with increasing age.

Sexual problems are also very common after a head injury, with approximately 50 per cent of people reporting some difficulty.

Common sexual problems after head injury

Men

Common sexual problems for men are listed in Table 8.1. There are medical treatments and sexual aids which may help. These aids can be purchased privately

Table 8.1 Common sexual problems for men after head injury

Problem	Treatment
Erectile dysfunction	
Difficulty attaining or maintaining an erection sufficient for intercourse. This can be caused by a variety of factors, such as disruption of the control by the brain, depression, or accompanying injuries to other parts of the body (e.g. the pelvis)	Oral medicines such as Viagra, Tadalis, and Cialis, which, taken prior to sexual activity, increase the likelihood of a good erection forming during sexual stimulation by dilating blood vessels in the penis, allowing blood to flow in to create the erection. Similar vasodilator drugs can be administered via the urethra or by injection into the side of the penis. There are also vacuum pump and constriction devices, which may be the treatment of choice for some
Ejaculation problems	
Difficulty in ejaculating can occur if there is not a firm enough erection for adequate stimulation of the penis, so that treatment of any erectile problem may resolve the ejaculatory problem. Sometimes this problem is separate from the erectile dysfunction	If the problem with ejaculation is due to inadequate stimulation of the penis because it is not firm enough, treatment of the erectile problem will resolve the ejaculation problem. If the ejaculatory delay is a separate problem the use of a vibrator may help

(see useful websites in Appendix 1). However, their use is often more successful when accompanied by advice and encouragement from a doctor or psychosexual therapist. The therapist would be able to assist the couple to talk about how these treatments can be incorporated into their sexual time together.

Women

Common sexual problems for women are listed in Table 8.2. As for men, there are treatments and helpful aids for women which can be prescribed or purchased. Again, discussion with a psychosexual therapist can be enabling and will provide a space to communicate any anxieties that the woman or her partner may have.

Men and women

Both men and women can experience other sexual difficulties.

◆ **Relationship problems** The impact of head injury on a relationship can be great and diverse. The changes in power and control that come with one partner becoming less mobile, unable to return to work or to care for the family, and dependent on their partner, perhaps even to help feed them or assist with personal care, are obvious. The injured person might wish to

Table 8.2 Common sexual problems for women after head injury

Problem	Treatment
Difficulties with arousal and orgasm	
This may be caused by sensory loss in the genital area, or feelings of shame if injuries have left any deformities	A vibrator can be very helpful in increasing genital stimulation and hence arousal
Painful intercourse	
This may be associated with lack of vaginal lubrication. If the woman is not becoming aroused because she does not feel sexual stimulation, she will not lubricate well. Fear of pain can cause spasm of the lower vaginal muscles, preventing easy penetration	If there is infection this must be treated by a doctor. Menopausal symptoms can often be managed with local oestrogen creams or hormone replacement therapy, as advised by a doctor. If there is vaginal dryness, lubricants applied before intercourse can make penetration much easier. Graded vaginal dilators used regularly and in sequence can help to relax the vaginal muscles and assist the woman to regain confidence until intercourse becomes comfortable again. It can be particularly useful to have the advice and encouragement of a psychosexual therapist when using dilators

resume sex quickly as it helps them to feel more powerful and able to do something for their partner again. However, you may find the switch from carer to lover more difficult and you may need more time to adjust. The partner who used to take the initiative sexually and was very active during foreplay and intercourse may have to accept a more passive role. Similarly, the partner who was used to taking a more passive role may have to become more active. These are major challenges and couples can feel deskilled at first and avoidance may seem easier than talking about it.

◆ **Loss of desire** This may be related to depression, anxiety, fatigue, low motivation, and hormonal changes (all of which can be experienced after head injury).

◆ **Difficulties in engaging in foreplay or getting into a comfortable position for intercourse** can also occur because of post-injury physical problems such as weakness or paralysis of limbs. Dealing with weakness or paralysis of limbs will require some creative thinking regarding comfortable positions for sexual activity and the use of pillows or other furniture.

◆ **Concerns over engaging in intercourse with a catheter** in place prevents many couples from trying. It is not impossible to have sexual intercourse with a catheter in place. Talking over anxieties with a doctor, nurse practitioner, or therapist may help to alleviate anxiety and help you to consider ways of managing.

◆ **Masturbation** In private this is a perfectly normal form of sexual behaviour. However, this can be very difficult for a man or woman who has weakness or paralysis of hands or arms. There is not always an easy solution to this, but the problem should not be ignored because it may be difficult to resolve.

◆ **Inappropriate behaviour** Because of the head injury, a person may unwittingly behave inappropriately; perhaps by talking too much and not listening, by moving too close to another making them feeling uncomfortable, or occasionally by speaking in a rude way, exposing sexual body areas, or touching another person's body inappropriately.

◆ **Worry about forming new relationships** Single head-injured people often worry about how they will meet partners in the future. This can be complicated if the person is living in residential care or with their parents, who might, understandably, find it difficult to balance caring for their child with allowing them privacy and opportunities to meet other young people who might become future partners. If the person with head injury had poor social skills prior to the injury, socializing afterwards can seem even more hazardous.

Causes of sexual problems after head injury

Sexual activity is complex and can be affected by many factors. Some of the post-injury physical factors (such as limb weakness) were mentioned in the previous section; however, psychological, emotional, and practical issues also have an important role in the development of sexual problems. Sexual problems after head injury rarely have a single cause.

Psychological factors

It is often the psychological or emotional changes that occur following head injury which interfere most profoundly with a person's ability to relate sexually. In particular, grief and loss, which are very much part of the normal recovery process for people with a head injury and their partners, can lead to poor self-esteem or even depression in both partners which will have a knock-on affect in the physical relationship.

Cognitive factors

Cognitive impairments such as loss of ability to initiate activities or to empathize with a partner can create major challenges for the injured person wanting to seek a partner or for the couple wanting to re-establish their sexual relationship.

Speech problems

Speech problems can also play a role in the development of sexual problems. Talking about personal issues is difficult enough, but trying to explain sexual desires, needs, or fears when there is a problem with understanding or expressing speech makes it even more difficult.

Pre-head injury factors

The relationship existing prior to the head injury also has a great impact on the development of the relationship after the injury.

- **Couples with a good relationship** prior to the injury, who had no major unresolved issues, who could communicate reasonably well, and who both wanted to be in the relationship will find that the trauma and consequent changes, although challenging, will probably not cause irreparable damage to the relationship. This couple may need to do some talking and readjusting, but will be able to do this with (or without) a little professional help. Sexually they may have anxieties and questions, but with information and encouragement they will move forward creatively together.

- In **couples with a troubled relationship** prior to the injury, who had many unresolved issues and found it very difficult to communicate or argued a lot when they tried, or where one or both partners may have been considering separation, the injury can bring all this sharply into focus. Often it is the partner of the injured person who is struggling with these issues before the injured person, who is initially very occupied with the recovery process. As this partner considers the future and his/her increased involvement with the injured partner, the pre-existing history of the relationship and buried issues and resentments surface and have to be dealt with. This is often a lonely time for the partner, who may not have access to all the help and encouragement that the injured partner is having. However, this can also be a frightening time for the injured partner, who may similarly be questioning the future of the relationship, but who also may be fearful that the alternatives to returning home may be equally challenging.

What can be done to help with sexual problems?

The cause of sexual problems is frequently multifactorial, and so psychological and relationship factors as well as the physical factors must be addressed for resolution to occur. Often, the biggest hurdle to finding ways of dealing with sexual difficulties is fear of talking about them with a partner or professional helper. If you can do this fairly early on, you are more likely to identify what the more important issues are and access the right kind of help.

Seek specialist counselling and advice

Referral to a specialist counsellor such as a relationship and psychosexual therapist is often very helpful. They can assist a couple to talk about their concerns, their relationship, and their sexual difficulties and help them understand what factors are contributing to their problems, enable them to express their fears, grief, and other feelings, and assist them to make decisions that are right for them and find creative ways forward. Accepting and adjusting to these changes involves some grieving in both partners. The changes in personality of the injured person and the roles of the couple can completely 'reshape' the relationship, generally and in the bedroom. If both partners have previously been independent and active people, giving each other a lot of emotional space, the increased dependency of one partner and the amount of time spent together after the brain injury can produce a strain on the couple and their relationship. Partners may equally experience a whole range of feelings including fear, anxiety, pity, shame, anger, helplessness, hopelessness, loneliness, and depression. This sort of input might be especially helpful for problems such as loss of desire which are usually caused by factors other than physical ones.

In addition, a speech and language therapist (SALT) may well be involved from the start of any rehabilitation programme assisting the head-injured person and his/her partner to communicate. A clinical psychologist may also be involved from early on in assessing cognitive ability and behaviour. He/she should be able to provide guidance with managing cognitive problems, mood changes, or any inappropriate behaviour.

Single people may also find time spent discussing their situation with a relationship and psychosexual therapist useful. A therapist may be accessed through Relate or the British Association for Sexual and Relationship Therapy (BASRT) (see websites in Appendix 1). Organizations such as Outsiders and Headway can help persons with head injury, who lack social skills and confidence, to practise socializing and make new friends.

Asking about medical treatments and useful aids

Any pre-existing medical conditions such as high blood pressure or diabetes must be monitored and managed by a medical professional. As medicines themselves may interfere with sexual functioning, it is important to review medication with your doctor.

Work with your partner and others to problem solve difficult situations

As we have stated throughout this book, it might also help to consider ways in which your environment can be adapted. Sometimes, where sex takes place is an issue, particularly if the injured partner cannot go upstairs to a double bed, or if she/he requires a special mattress and has a single bed. Often difficulties with dressing and undressing produce new challenges for a couple. Being able to talk together about these things creates opportunities for solutions to be found. Again, a psychosexual therapist can help the couple to talk more easily.

❓ Frequently asked questions

Is the sexual problem my relative has permanent and is there treatment for it?

If the sexual problems have been caused by your relative's head injury, there may be recovery of function along with the recovery of other physical functions. If the problem is permanent, there are physical treatments and medicines for some sexual problems and your GP or your relative's neurological rehabilitation doctor may be able to advise you. If the problem arises mainly because of psychological or relationship issues following the injury, a psychosexual therapist could help you both work on these issues. If the sexual problem is permanent, the therapist can assist you and your partner to be creative and adapt to these changes.

With the disabilities that my relative has, how will they meet a partner in the future?

Even without the disabilities associated with head injury, meeting a partner can be a challenge. It depends on so many factors including personality, opportunity, experience of mixing with people, and past experiences of relationships. When you also have physical and/or cognitive disabilities, the challenge is even greater. Finding opportunities to meet other people, develop confidence, and practice social skills can be enhanced by organizations such as Headway and Outsiders. Talking to a relationship and psychosexual therapist can help your relative think about his/her experiences of and concerns about mixing with people and making relationships.

Where can I find information about sexual problems and the right professionals to help?

Useful resources are listed in Appendix 1. You can also talk about this to your GP or your relative's neurorehabilitation doctor. They may give you information/links to useful organizations.

9

Family issues after head injury

 Key points

- Head injury can have a significant emotional impact on the whole family, not just the injured person.

- A wide range of emotional reactions can be experienced by relatives—there is no 'typical' response and no right or wrong way to feel.

- Families have a wide range of information and support needs at all stages of the recovery process.

- Useful family coping strategies include:

  - becoming knowledgeable about head injury

  - learning how to support the injured relative

  - seeking support from others in the same situation and sharing experiences.

So far we have focused on the wide-ranging effects of head injury on the injured person. However, head injury is a crisis which affects not just the injured person, but all members of the family. It is now well recognized that its impact can be as devastating, if not more so, for the relatives as it is for the patient him/herself.

Focusing on family issues is important because:

- head injury can cause family members themselves to experience significant distress, often to the extent that they warrant treatment and help in their own right

- families play a major role in helping people recover from head injury yet the distress they experience can interfere with this.

Therefore, in this chapter we turn our attention to helping you:

- understand the possible impact of your relative's head injury on you and your family

- develop ways to cope.

As we have stated throughout the book, not all families have the same needs or face the same problems; also, not all the strategies listed here work for everyone.

We have structured the information around **the key tasks and challenges facing families throughout the head injury 'journey'** (as outlined in Chapter 2). We have been careful to avoid trying to categorize these challenges into specific time phases after the injury as it is our experience that many of these issues arise in an unpredictable way, occurring time after time for some families, or not at all for others.

The key tasks and challenges facing families after head injury

- Understanding and making sense of head injury and hospital systems.
- Dealing with their own fears, worries, and emotional reactions to the injury.
- Coping with the changed relative.
- Adjusting to family role and relationship changes.
- Managing the common post-injury practical problems.
- Supporting other family members and friends in dealing with the crisis.

Making sense of head injury and hospital systems

Research has shown that families have extensive **information needs** after a relative's head injury, and when these are not addressed they can feel less able to cope. Family information needs tend to focus on:

- needing to understand more about the nature of the relative's brain injury, how it occurred, its effects, its prognosis, and options for treatment
- being clear about the pathway of care that the relative might follow and knowing how to navigate around the hospital system
- needing to have clear ongoing information at times of key transitions (e.g. information about discharge and further treatment options).

Therefore a useful starting point in the very early stages following the accident is to seek as much **information** as possible about your relative's condition (this is also discussed in Chapter 1). Useful sources of information include Headway, the hospital's Head Injury Nurse (if there is one) and your relative's care manager (if one has been appointed–this is usually a hospital social worker). Your local Headway group may also have access to a Family Support Worker. There are also many excellent websites that provide general introductory facts about head injury (see Appendix 1).

The need for information continues throughout the recovery process. Chapter 3 takes you through various pathways of care that head-injured people may follow which take some of the confusion out of the 'maze' of services. For those who have enjoyed a good recovery, longer-term information needs will most likely focus on issues such as returning to work, driving, and resuming leisure activities (these are discussed in Chapter 11).

Understanding and managing your emotional reactions

> 'It's a juggling act. . . a rollercoaster of emotions. One day you're down, the next you're back up again; you constantly have to balance positive feelings against your fears and as my relative is changing all the time so are my emotions. . .'

No two head injuries are ever the same; similarly no two families are the same. Therefore it follows that your experience of head injury will be different from that of other families. To complicate matters further, the reactions among your own relatives are also likely to vary, perhaps depending on how close they are to the injured person or the type of relationship they have with them. However, there *are* reactions and emotions that are shared by all.

Extensive research has focused on how families react emotionally to head injury in a close relative. This concludes the following.

- Family members experience a wide array of emotions and reactions after head injury as they try to cope with the challenges associated with it—all of these are *normal*.

- Typically, there is an episodic quality to these reactions, with families finding themselves re-experiencing similar emotions at different points in time. For example, a family might expeience great shock when their relative is first injured, but as they stabilize this changes to a sense of hope. However, when the patient later experiences a setback the family are plunged back into the shock and anxiety that they had felt in the very early stages of the crisis. The reoccurrence of earlier emotions can be unexpected and can lead families to feel as if they are not moving forward emotionally.

- These emotional reactions can be significant for many people and they may require professional help.

- The emotional strain of having a head-injured relative can worsen, rather than lessen, with time. This is particularly the case when families are dealing with a relative's severe behavioural and cognitive problems.

◆ It is not all bad. Not everyone experiences significant problems after a relative's head injury, and for many it brings a new and more positive focus to the family.

❌ **Myth** Some researchers have suggested that the process of adjusting to a relative's head injury follows a series of predictable distinct stages, each expected at particular time points following the injury. It is suggested that relatives can expect initially to feel emotions such as shock, then pass through other reactions such as anger, and finally, with the passing of time, reach acceptance of the injury.

❗ **Fact** Many families *will* share similar emotional reactions. However, it is too simplistic to see the process of adjusting to head injury as following a simple predictable pattern. Some families will not experience all possible reactions and some will experience certain emotional reactions at times much later or earlier than other families. It is also possible for families to pass through some stages, or experience emotional reactions such as anger, more than once. We have learned that the process of coming to terms with a relative's injuries is a dynamic ever-changing one that shifts not just with time, but also in response to what is happening in the lives of the injured person and their families.

A wide range of reactions is possible after a relative's head injury—there is no right or wrong, good or bad way to react. It is important to let your feelings come naturally and not to feel troubled if your way of responding is not the same as the reactions of others in the family.

Emotional shock

Most people are emotionally *shocked* at the news that their relative has been injured. Shock can affect people in different ways: some people show their emotions outwardly (e.g. crying or shouting) while others appear to remain calm and in control. Some people can seem unaffected by the news they have just been given. However, for them, and others, things may feel unreal. When in shock, it is hard to take in or remember information that is given, and you can find yourself asking the same questions over and over. It can help to ask for written information from staff if this is the case.

Emotional numbness

Emotional numbness is a common early reaction to trauma (and can also be seen following bereavement). You feel as if you have lost your ability to feel emotions and you may feel 'numb' or 'frozen' emotionally. Many people describe feeling unable to act or do anything (like a 'rabbit caught in the headlights'). This can be a disturbing sensation as it may make you feel distant from others, who may be expressing their feelings more openly. However, other people find that being on this emotional 'auto-pilot' can help them to cope.

Guilt

As the news of the relative's injury sinks in, families are commonly affected by feelings of *guilt*, when they can believe *irrationally* that there was something they could have done to have prevented it from happening. Children in families are very vulnerable to feeling as if they could have caused the injury (i.e. through being naughty or causing stress). Guilt can result in family members feeling that they have to 'make up' for what has happened and protect the relative from further harm. This can lead to conflict or can limit the injured person's confidence and increase their dependence on others.

What helps to manage guilt?

- Acknowledge that feelings of guilt are common.
- Do not play the 'What if?' game (e.g. 'What if I had been driving instead of him. . .') as this is only likely to increase your distress.
- Do not torture yourself over things that were said (or not said) to the injured person before the accident. People often regret and can become preoccupied with thoughts that they did not say 'goodbye' properly the last time they saw the person, that they did not tell them that they love them, or that an argument had not been resolved. This is just part of everyday life and no one can prepare for such situations. Counselling might help to explore strong and disabling feelings of guilt that continue long term.
- Work closely with therapists involved with your relative to help you step back and allow the injured person to take some risks safely. It is often easier to 'let go' when we are supported to do so.

Denial

In the early stages it is not unusual for families to find it hard to accept or believe the information they have been given about their loved one (e.g. that their relative might die). This reaction is sometimes referred to as *denial* and is common when people are given bad news (it is experienced to an extent by almost everyone). There is an assumption that denial is not a helpful reaction, but this is too simplistic. What seems to be important is the stage at which denial is used. In the acute stages of a crisis, denial can help keep people 'going', not 'fall apart' and therefore it is seen as useful. However, denial in the later stages of the recovery process, particularly in the longer term, has been shown to be problematic for most families and injured people, particularly as it can be accompanied by unrealistic expectations. When these expectations are not met there can be strong feelings of disappointment, failure, and hopelessness.

Denial may also result in families failing to acknowledge the reasons for changes in the injured person (e.g. it may be difficult to understand and accept that aggressive behaviours are occurring because of the direct results of permanent damage to the brain). Importantly, denial can interfere with families being able to seek the appropriate types of help and can contribute to prolonged or delayed emotional stress.

What can help with denial?

◆ Work closely with your relative's therapists to receive regular, honest, and realistic feedback on their progress. This will help you acknowledge and understand their strengths and weaknesses and to start to appraise your situation in light of this.

◆ Take one day at a time—allow difficult information to 'sink in' gradually.

◆ Share your feelings and experiences with others at family or carers support groups.

Anxiety

Families can experience high levels of fear and anxiety after head injury, especially in the early stages if they are unsure whether their relative will survive. This time of waiting can cause great strain, with many families feeling extreme distress as they try to cope with the uncertainty. Sudden and unpredictable bouts of crying are common at this time, as are loss of appetite, sleeplessness, and a sense of agitation and feeling as if you need to do something. These feelings tend to lessen as more information is gained about the relative's prospects or as they start to show signs of early recovery. However, for some people anxiety can continue to be problematic in the long term and can be very disabling.

Helpful strategies

◆ Allow yourself a time each day to focus on your worries; try to write them down or talk them over with someone. Next, make plans to deal with the issues that can be tackled quickly. Following this, try to keep busy and focused on other activities, to distract yourself, and to avoid being overwhelmed by problems that you have not yet tackled.

◆ Try to work on preventing a build-up of stress as it can have a negative effect on your physical and emotional health. Make time each day for relaxation. There are many ways in which to do this including simply sitting quietly, listening to music, attending a yoga class, or taking part in physical activity such as swimming or walking (you may need to arrange for someone to be with your relative while you are busy).

◆ Learning to relax can be difficult, especially when you are under stress, and so it might help to attend a relaxation class. Ask at your GP practice or the library for details of what is available in your area. You could also borrow DVDs, CDs, and books from your local library that teach relaxation skills.

◆ Try to remember that you will support your relative more effectively if you take time to care for yourself and manage your stress.

Anger and frustration

Anger is common after head injury. It can be a very powerful emotion and is often justified but it can interfere with being able to think clearly and rationally. Anger may be directed towards the following:

◆ Others involved in the accident or who might have caused the injury, and this anger may be accompanied by a strong desire to seek revenge. Teenagers in families can be particularly vulnerable to such thoughts (see Chapter 10).

◆ The injured person—this may take you by surprise and be hard to admit.

◆ Medical staff, especially if families feel that their relative is not receiving the right kind of treatment or when families are not provided with adequate information, which can exacerbate feelings of helplessness and confusion. Families are often frustrated by how often they are given the response 'We don't know' in answer to their questions (especially about prognosis and longer-term outcome). While it can be very difficult to feel as if no one is giving you clear answers, it might help to know that 'We don't know' is often the most appropriate answer to early questions.

◆ Some people do not know where to direct their emotions and simply feel angry with the world or with a 'higher power', such as God. Previously held religious (and other) beliefs can be challenged and the world can feel as it is an unsafe and insecure place.

Anger can be experienced at all stages in the recovery process. It can re-emerge or be re-triggered at times of heightened emotional distress (such as during court proceedings about the accident).

What can help?

◆ Anger typically occurs when communication breaks down and people feel that they are not being listened to. Seek information, and ensure that you have enough support and that you feel you are being heard.

◆ Try not to suppress angry thoughts or push them aside (which can increase stress); instead try to accept them as a 'normal' part of coming to terms with what has happened. Promise yourself that you will not act on these feelings until the 'crisis' has passed and you have had time to think things through.

Emotional relief

Relief is also a common reaction, often in the early stages. Being told that your relative is stable and unlikely to die is usually accompanied by overwhelming relief and a sense of gratefulness. Often families let their guard down a little at this point and may experience a surge of emotions that have previously been held in check; this is normal but may be unexpected and overwhelming. Emotional relief can trigger high (possibly unrealistic) hope and expectations of full recovery.

Depression

Persistent feelings of sadness, despair, and hopelessness (that do not pass) are among the most common longer-term problems reported by family members. Depression is often accompanied by loss of enjoyment of things, lack of energy, poor sleep, and increased tearfulness. There can also be feelings of being overwhelmed by the situation and feeling unable to cope. It is more than feeling 'down' or 'a bit low'. Depression tends to develop in tandem with the gradual realization that the relative is unlikely to recover, which can be particularly difficult after the initial period of hope and optimism that may have been felt in the early stages of recovery. Research suggests that many family members rely on medication (such as antidepressants, tranquillizers, and sleep medications) to help them cope with depression after a relative's head injury. Symptoms of depression include:

- problems sleeping
- poor self-care
- extreme guilt
- feeling completely alone
- excessive use of alcohol or drugs
- feeling hopeless about the future
- possible thoughts of suicide or self-harming.

What can help?

- Take symptoms of depression seriously and seek help. See your GP immediately and be guided by him/her. He/she may suggest a trial of medication and/or counselling.

- Set realistic achievable goals for yourself and your relative.

- Try to pay attention to how you are thinking about (appraising) your relative's injury and what it means for you. It is easy to feel overwhelmed when thinking about the enormity and uncertainty of the changes you are facing—some people liken it to facing an enormous wall that has to be knocked over in 'one go'. Instead, it may be helpful to try to see the head injury as triggering many smaller changes that you have to get used to and adjust to. This way you will be knocking the wall down brick by brick, making the task seem a little easier.

- Go easy on yourself—try to be mindful of when you use terms such as 'should' and 'must' (e.g. 'I must telephone all our relatives today to let them know how John is progressing') as these can make you feel under pressure. Instead try to tell yourself: 'It would be nice if I could let the family know how John is doing. I will phone as many people as I am able to. The others will understand if I don't get around to them today.'

- Seek the company and support of family and close friends.

Grief

The emotional reactions associated with head injury have been likened to the feelings experienced by families following bereavement. While some of the responses felt after head injury may be similar to those felt after a relative's death (such as loss, despair, sadness), there are some quite distinct differences. Head injury tends to result in an *incomplete* grief reaction as the person, who has been changed (but not killed) by the head injury, is only partially lost—they look the same but are different. As many post-injury changes are permanent, few families will experience the final closure to this grief that death can bring.

What can help?

- Allow yourself to grieve.
- Discuss and share these feelings with other family members.
- Seek counselling.
- Attend a family support group.
- Set realistic limits for your relative—acknowledge that they have changed and may not be able to achieve what they could have before. This helps to reduce disappointment and further feelings of sadness and loss. Concentrating on your relative's strengths will help you to take a more positive focus.

Acceptance

It is often assumed that the process of family emotional adjustment results in a final stage of acceptance. However, although this is the case for many families, it does not necessarily imply a positive acceptance. For some people, acceptance is synonymous with 'giving up' or 'giving in' to the head injury, and with losing their sense of hope and fight. Acceptance may be accompanied by a re-emergence of both sadness and anger as families are required to find a new way of living. Acceptance of the injury and its effects is less problematic for other families, and they are able to move on positively. As such, the notion of acceptance can hold both positive and negative meanings for families.

Positive personal growth

Despite the difficulties discussed here, there is evidence that families can, over time, report positive outcomes from traumatic experiences such as head injury. Positive effects include increased family closeness, enhanced ability to cope with stress, recognition of their personal strength, appreciation of life, and spiritual development.

What can help manage troublesome emotional reactions?

Many of the early reactions described above dissipate as more clarity and understanding about the injured person's condition and prospects are gained. Support from others can also be helpful. The two main types we recommend are counselling and family support groups.

Counselling

Many family members feel the need to seek more formal emotional support, such as counselling. Counselling involves the opportunity to meet regularly with a professional who is trained to listen to and support people who may be in crisis and need help to get through a difficult life event. It is usually time limited (e.g. perhaps for six weekly sessions) and offers you the chance to explore issues that may be concerning or distressing you.

Counselling provides families with a safe and confidential opportunity to discuss feelings of personal responsibility for their relative's illness (especially common in the early stages), loss of control, guilt or fear about the future, and distressing thoughts (such as wishing that the injured person had died) so that they can move on from these reactions, reduce the distress associated with them, and be able to start functioning effectively in everyday life. Counselling can also be helpful when needing to work through difficult decisions following the injury (such as deciding to separate from the injured person). It can also provide the opportunity to develop techniques for changing how you think about and manage the situations facing you.

Options for counselling will vary according to where you live but may be sought via the following:

◆ Your GP surgery: some GPs have access to counsellors within the practice. They are not likely to be specialists in head injury but will still be able to support you through the experience. Alternatively, your GP may be able to access specialist counsellors if you have a neurorehabilitation facility in your area.

◆ Your local branch of Headway may also have access to (or could fund) counsellors (who are likely to have more experience of working with the relatives of head-injured people). Headway family support workers can also offer a 'listening ear' but may not have formal counselling training.

◆ If your relative is in a rehabilitation facility, there may be various forms of family emotional support available there, including counsellors and clinical psychologists. Speak to your relative's primary nurse in the first instance.

◆ Counselling can also be accessed privately (see www.babcp.org for details of counsellors).

Some families find it useful to seek help from their own, or the hospital, chaplain/spiritual advisor. For those who prefer to seek more 'anonymous' forms of help, the Samaritans (tel: 08457 909090) may be an option.

Family support groups

Many families find support groups helpful after head injury. They can provide:

◆ an opportunity to discuss head-injury-related problems and the chance to learn from the experience of others

◆ emotional support and a safe place to vent difficult feelings

- relief from stress
- strategies for different ways of coping
- information
- a way to reduce isolation and provide an opportunity to expand social networks.

Local branches of Headway often provide support groups, and many people consider them a 'lifeline'.

If you do not wish to attend physically a support group, you could take part in newsgroups on the Internet dedicated to brain injury (try typing 'brain injury newsgroup' into Internet search engines such as Yahoo and Google). This will give you online support and chat with other people affected by head injury at a time that is convenient to you (and with anonymity if you require it).

Coping with changes in your relative

A major source of stress (often referred to as a 'burden') for relatives in the later stages of recovery are the ongoing changes in emotional control, personality, or behaviour in the injured person (discussed in Chapter 7).

What can help?

- Acknowledge and try to accept that almost all head-injured people 'change' to some extent after their accident.

- Share the experience with others who have first-hand experience of this problem. Carers support groups might be helpful or you might consider seeking counselling with a specialist head injury counsellor.

- Work closely with your relative's therapists to learn practical ways of coping with and managing changes. Try to focus your efforts on what can be changed and adjusting to what cannot be changed.

- It is helpful to remember that your relative is likely to change further as recovery continues. Some family members, having adjusted to the initial change brought about by the head injury, can have trouble 'letting go' and learning to be less protective towards their relative as they begin to show signs of improvement. This can lead to family stress and tension (especially around issues of risk-taking, such as the injured person wishing to resume driving again but the family worrying about safety), and professional support and advice may be needed to resolve this. Similarly, families have often put their own lives 'on hold' while their relative is recovering and tell us that they no longer feel needed or useful, which is also distressing.

- Families whose relatives remain very impaired after treatment (e.g. continue to experience severe problems with cognition, control of emotion or behaviour) are typically in greatest need of support (especially if the injured person returns home). This can be the time when 'reality' sinks in and the challenges of living with a head-injured person become clearer. In such instances families may need specialist advice and practical support, such as seeking day care or respite for their relative. Research has shown that one of the most helpful things for families is social support, and so it is important to enlist the help of family and friends, where possible. Your local Carers Centre is also a useful source of practical advice and emotional support (see www. carers.org.uk).

Adjusting to family role and relationship changes

People with head injury typically experience a loss of their previous roles within the family. This may mean that they no longer have the same responsibilities or undertake the same duties within the family (and everyday life) as they did before the injury; for example, someone who went out to work full time and was the main 'breadwinner' may now not be able to work. This can have an impact on other members of the family who might need to take on these roles instead.

There might also be changes in the quality and intensity of family relationships and alterations in the ways in which family members interact with and relate to each other. This might include changes in the way you communicate, problem-solve, and deal with issues. These changes may be very hard to manage. When these role and relationship changes endure, are very marked, or are inadequately managed, relationship problems can occur (in many cases resulting in separation and/or divorce, the rates of which are much higher in people with head injury than in the general population).

However, relationship difficulties are not inevitable. Post-injury changes can be positive for some families, with the injury resulting in them spending more time together, and achieving a better understanding and appreciation of each other (head injury is often said to put life 'into perspective' for families).

What can help?

Learning to adjust to changes within the family is rarely easy.

◆ Accept that role changes are almost inevitable after head injury.

◆ Try not to make irreversible decisions based on early role changes too soon in the recovery process (e.g. selling the family business because it is thought that the injured person will never resume their work role). Only make these decisions when you have as much information as possible, have talked them through with key people involved, and you feel that your own stress is well managed.

◆ Keeping a diary/journal can be helpful. It can provide an outlet for expressing worries and concerns, and it can be looked at later to help you see how things have changed (it is easy to lose perspective).

◆ Develop a plan with the injured person (aided by a health care professional) to help them gradually to resume some of their previous roles (even if just in part).

◆ Family sessions with trained professionals can be used to address changes in relationships or ways of communicating in the family that are very troublesome. Work with families can include formal family therapy (a structured psychological intervention undertaken by specially trained therapists and usually offered to target specific significant family difficulties). However, most families do not require family therapy, but may benefit from family sessions (with head injury professionals) during which issues of concern can be addressed. Such sessions are typically offered by clinical neuropsychologists but may also be with social workers, counsellors, or doctors. Ask your GP, Headway, or your local head injury team about what is available.

Managing practical problems

Many practical problems can arise following head injury, such as financial concerns (e.g. you may have less money coming into the household if your injured relative is no longer able to work), accessibility issues (e.g. needing to consider moving from your home if it cannot be adapted to suit your relative's physical problems), or transport problems, all of which can contribute to family stress. Families may also have to cope with loss of support from the extended family and friends over time, and as a result may become socially and emotionally isolated, and feel stigmatized and lonely (which in turn can worsen their distress). Having fewer people to turn to for help can seem to exacerbate many practical problems.

What can help?

◆ Seek advice from your local carers centre or branch of Headway on practical support that might be available to you. Dialability (a national charity offering advice on equipment and aids) can also be a useful source of advice.

◆ Feeling unable to socialize often arises from other difficult emotions such as anger and hopelessness. It can be helpful to talk these through (with friends, family, or a counsellor) and try to find ways round them.

◆ Attend a family/relatives support group (see above).

◆ Increase social competence by going out and facing people, even when it feels difficult to do so—to avoid social withdrawal. Plan outings with people who can support you.

◆ Seek support from outside the family.

◆ Try to maintain (or re-activate) your previous contacts, friendships, and activities as far as possible. Tell them as much as you and your relative are comfortable with about the injury and its consequences so that they can understand your situation.

◆ Think carefully about whether you should give up your own work and only do so if it is really necessary.

Supporting other family members and friends

It is helpful to seek and accept the support of those that you are close to. However, it is important to remember that head injury can also have an emotional effect on both close and extended family, and also on friends and work colleagues. Those outside the immediate family may find it difficult to access information about the injured person's status and progress, and, like the average person, they are unlikely to know much about head injury. As a result, they may feel very worried and confused about what is going on and may choose to contact you for information. Managing requests for updates, progress reports, and information from others can be a significant source of stress for the injured person's immediate family (especially in the very early days post-injury), as is managing the distress of others.

What can help?

- Nominate a reliable family member as the key family communication person, whom friends and relatives should be directed to contact for information instead of you. Alternatively, this 'newslink' person could send regular updates to family and friends by e-mail or text.

- Draw up a timetable for family and friends to visit your relative. This will ensure that your relative always has enough visitors (but not too many, to avoid 'overload') and may enable you to leave them for short periods.

- Set clear ground rules for visits. These should be based on what you and the injured person need and want. For example, some families agree that they will not cry in front of the injured person or that only positive issues can be discussed at the bedside. There are no right and wrong answers to this issue, but whatever is agreed should be communicated clearly to all involved and adhered to consistently.

A source of stress for many families during the post-acute stage is managing advice from family and friends. During the acute (early) phase there is a greater tendency for families to listen to the advice of the professionals (because of the immediacy of medical problems). However, as time passes family members often start to develop their own ideas about the injured person's problems and may begin to offer you advice (much of which is likely to be conflicting).

What can help?

- It is advisable to listen carefully to all advice given, but not to act on it until you have given it careful thought.

- Try to be assertive and tell others when you do not want to receive advice or help. It can be difficult to do this without them feeling criticized or offended, but can be easier for them to accept if you are able to tell them what would help you instead.

◆ Ultimately it is important to deal with issues in the way that you and your injured relative are happy with; try not to be too concerned with what others think.

Close friends (especially of the injured person) can play an important role in their recovery but they will also need help coming to terms with what has happened.

What can help?

◆ Try to be patient with friends, especially when they do not seem to understand your relative's problems. It can help to remember that, as you spend much more time with your relative, their difficulties are likely to be more familiar to you.

◆ Take time to explain the injury and its effects to close friends so that they understand what your relative needs. Encourage them to pass on this information to other friends.

◆ Give friends a distinct role if possible. They are usually keen to help but may not know what is needed (e.g. could they drive the injured person to their weekly speech therapy appointment?)

◆ Encourage them, as far as possible, to maintain the interests that they previously shared with the injured person (e.g. continue playing golf together). This will help your relative maintain some continuity with the past, provide them with a 'normal' social outlet, and may give other family members some much needed time without them.

Special issues for different family members

Most family members experience similar concerns and issues after a relative's head injury but, depending on their relationship with the injured person, there may be particular issues that perhaps no one in the family shares with them.

Understanding spouses' issues

The spouses and partners of people with head injury have probably received most of the research attention when families have been the subject of studies. The special issues for them include the following:

◆ Dealing with the 'loss' of their life partner (and shared life plans), their sexual partner, and, if there are children in the family, their co-parent. It may be difficult for other family members to appreciate fully the extent of the losses felt.

◆ Coping with taking on new roles and responsibilities within the family. This might include having to become the main earner (especially stressful for spouses who did not work previously) or having to assume unfamiliar roles (e.g. a mother may have to assume the injured father's previous role of taking the children to football practice). Spouses may also become the injured person's main carer, which can have a significant impact on their relationship. In particular, taking on carer duties is often accompanied by loss of the sexual relationship, especially when a spouse feels that they now have a parental rather than marital relationship with their partner. Care-taking commitments can also result in spouses sacrificing their own needs (e.g. giving up their career or social life) in favour of those of the injured partner. This can lead to a reduced quality of life for spouses.

◆ Spouses may feel trapped inside the marriage following the injury. They may want to separate from the partner but feel unable to because of a sense of duty, guilt, and fear of being negatively judged by other family members and professionals. Unfortunately, the rate of relationship breakdown after a head injury is high (significantly higher than in the general population)—counselling may be useful in such situations.

◆ When there are dependent children in the family, spouses may also feel addi-tional strain in supporting their injured partner in their ongoing parental role. They may have concerns about their partner's ability to carry out this role (perhaps because of cognitive problems) but be unsure how to address or access support (the issues around parenting after head injury are still not ade-quately addressed by most head injury services). Spouses may find themselves drawn into a clash of loyalties, wishing to support their partner's parental role and authority within the family, yet at the same time wishing to safeguard their children's well-being. When risk issues emerge (e.g. in relation to children's safety), people are often afraid to seek help from outside agencies for fear of stigma and serious consequences for their partner and children.

Parents of injured adult children

Parents whose adult children are head injured also face some potentially unique challenges, especially if their child has a partner or spouse. Clashes can occur between the two parties on how the injured person should be managed and cared for, and in some cases this can lead to tension and breakdown in relationships. Some parents wish to care for their injured 'child' themselves, but this might undermine the injured person's spouse, who may be struggling to accept this role, or who might wish for their partner to be cared for elsewhere. However, some parents may not wish to resume such a role as it may interfere with their plans (e.g. to retire abroad) and may resent any expectations that professionals may have for them to do so.

It can help if all involved parties meet with one of the injured person's therapists to talk through how these types of situations can be managed.

Close friends of the injured person

Head injury can affect all the people that are connected to the injured person, including friends. Friends are likely to experience the wide range of emotional reactions described earlier, such as shock, fear, and anger, but are less likely to be offered support from services and so may struggle to understand and manage their reactions.

Friends can also experience some degree of role change in relation to the injured person, which they will have to adapt to. They may have to take on a more supervisory role, help the person practically more than they used to (e.g. make meals for them), or become involved in aspects of their care (e.g. assisting with toilet use when out on a day trip). While friends might welcome the opportunity to help and willingly take on these new roles, the nature of their relationship with the injured person will undoubtedly change as result. In many cases relationships and emotional bonds are strengthened, but others can become strained and friendships are lost.

Children with head injured relatives

Children with head injured relatives have wide-ranging needs, especially when the injured relative is their parent. This is discussed in Chapter 10.

 Questions frequently asked by relatives

- **Will I feel better over time?**

    Because of the unique nature of head injury we cannot predict how you and your family will feel in the future. While we know that many families find positive aspects to their lives many years after head injury, for some families there is a trend for their emotional problems to worsen over time, and this is particularly the case when the injured relative has ongoing behavioural and emotional problems. Therefore, if this is one of your relative's primary issues, it is important to seek help now—for them and for support for you and your family in coping with them.

- **Why do other families that we have met seem to be reacting so differently from us to their relative's head injury?**

    How a family responds to and deals with a relative's head injury depends on many different factors.

    - How each family functions (both before and after the injury—all families have their particular ways of dealing with problems and rising to challenges).

    - The quality and closeness of famly relationships (some families are emotionally closer than others).

    - The effects of the head injury itself (you will remember reading earlier that families often find it harder to cope with marked changes in their relative's behaviour).

◆ The type and amount of help the family receives (from professionals and from family and friends—the more support the better!).

◆ Other family problems: it is important to remember that the problems families might be experiencing can arise because of the general stress of having a relative who is ill, or the strain associated with some of the challenging problems your relative might be experiencing. For other families, issues may reflect a worsening or triggering of problems that existed before the accident.

Given this wide range of possibilities it becomes easier to see why no two families' experience of head injury will ever be very similar.

◆ **Should we hide our feelings from our injured relative as we are afraid it will make them worse?**

There is no right or wrong answer to this question and you, as a family, should do what you think will work best for you all. Are you a family who have always openly shown and shared your emotions? If so, your relative is likely to notice any changes to this and might become suspicious or afraid of why people are acting differently towards them. They may be anxious that you are all hiding something dreadful. It is generally always better to try to be open and honest with each other and to share your feelings and concerns. However, some head-injured people find coping with emotions (especially those of others) difficult and so may either become overwhelmed by your distress or be unable to respond to it and seem indifferent. Seek the advice of a clinical neuropsychologist about useful ways of sharing concerns with your relative. Ensure that you have a support network among family and friends so that you do not need to rely solely on the injured person for support at this time.

10

Helping children cope with head injury in the family

 Key points

- Children, like adults, are affected emotionally when a close relative, especially a parent, is head injured.

- They need honest age-appropriate information to help them understand head injury, and an opportunity to express feelings and concerns. Sometimes counselling may be necessary.

- Children (of all ages) can feel that they are to blame for the injury and need to be reassured about this.

- There is a link between the ways that children and adults cope with stressful events. It helps if adults can model positive coping strategies for the younger members of the family.

- Head injury services do not routinely offer support to children, so adults need to be proactive about asking for help.

In this chapter we turn our attention to the issues faced by children who have a close relative, particularly a parent, with head injury. We discuss the ways in which children can be affected by family head injury and provide guidance for adults on how to explain head injury and support children.

We have written this as a separate chapter for the following reasons.

- Children have their own special needs at times of stress and cannot be regarded as 'mini-adults'.

- Head injury services do not routinely offer help to children (because of lack of resources, lack of expertise, and lack of awareness of the issues facing them). However, without advice, it can be difficult for families to know how best to help children through this emotional experience. It is hoped that this chapter will address this gap and increase your confidence in supporting children and asking for help for them at this difficult time.

The information contained here is directed, in the main, towards helping children who have a head-injured parent. However, much of it is applicable to children with other relatives with head injury, such as a grandparent or a sibling. We provide guidance on children's information and support needs at the different stages of their relative's recovery, and as children's needs also vary with age, we have tried to draw out the key issues for children at various ages. This might be helpful to families where there are children with different age ranges.

How are children affected by head injury in the family?

The challenges and tasks faced by children when a parent (or other close relative) is injured are, in the main, very similar to those experienced by the adults in the family (e.g. having to cope with the changed relative, managing role and relationship changes). However, the implications of these challenges for children, and how they are experienced and understood by them, are different from the implications for adults.

- Because of their age and lack of life experience, children may find it much harder than adults to comprehend or make sense of the changes observed in the parent. In particular, children (often secretly) worry that they might have caused their parent's injury in some way.

- Witnessing such changes (especially cognitive and behavioural changes) can affect how children go on to develop emotionally. Infants and toddlers, especially, can be confused, unsettled, and afraid of the altered parent; this can affect the bond or attachment they had with that parent and can make them feel insecure. As a result, they may become very unsettled, and not recognize or know how to relate to the 'new' parent.

- Role changes within the family can also impact on children. Even very young children may be required to assume additional household duties to try to support the uninjured parent who may be caring for their spouse. Older children may be given extra responsibility, perhaps being asked to look after younger children in the family. They may be asked to 'keep an eye' on the injured person and this can gradually reverse roles, where children become almost parent-like towards the adult. This has been shown to have detrimental effects for both children and adults, even though most children will willingly take on the role of '**young carer**'. Very young children might have their place as 'the baby' in the family taken from them by a very needy injured parent, leaving them feeling neglected or ignored.

- Children may be 'stigmatized' for having a parent who is 'different' and may be teased or bullied at school. Teachers may be unaware of the potential impact of head injury on families, and may be oblivious to the issues facing children or how to help them. Again, children may not openly discuss these problems for fear of causing additional family stress. Instead, they may try to resolve these issues alone, or 'act them out' in the form of problematic behaviour or poor school performance.

- Children, like adults, also suffer the effects of the problems that can arise following head injury, such as financial difficulties, relationship breakdown, and house moves. However, unlike adults, they are often less emotionally equipped to cope with such issues and may worry only about how they will be personally affected. Older children may alter their own life plans in response to the changed family circumstances; for example, teenagers do not apply to universities far from home (as previously planned) as they feel that they must stay close to the family. However, this is often accompanied by feelings of resentment.

- Children's ability to cope with the changed family life is also limited by the lack of information and support available to them (therefore we have provided some brief information that you might want to read with your children in Appendices 2 and 3).

- Children can also be affected further by the reduced physical and emotional availability of the non-injured parent, who is likely to be preoccupied with their partner's needs, or who may be too distressed themselves to be able to acknowledge their children's needs.

The small amount of research that has been carried out tells us that, when faced with these challenges, children can experience many of the problems that adults face, including anxiety, worry, depression, fear, and embarrassment. In addition, children of different ages tend to react in different ways (which might, if you have children of different ages in your family, explain why they could each be exhibiting different types of problems).

- **Babies and infants** (who are often mistakenly thought not to be affected by events going on around them because they cannot yet comprehend them) tend to show problems such as unsettled behaviour, disturbed sleep, and feeding difficulties at times of family stress.

- **Pre-schoolers** can become clingy (because they feel insecure), may have more temper tantrums, and may lose some of their previously acquired skills (e.g. begin bed-wetting again). They may also develop new fears (e.g. of the dark).

- **School-age children (pre-teens)** worry about being different from their friends and are vulnerable to being teased about their parent being 'odd'. They may become sad and withdrawn and fall behind in their school work. They can also show an increase in fears and phobias (in particular, they can fear others in the family coming to harm).

- **Teenagers** may respond with resentment and anger. They might also become tired (as a result of having to take on additional household tasks) and their schoolwork could suffer. They may show an increase in mood swings and oppositional behaviour (this is often characteristic of 'normal' teenage years anyway) and stay out of the house and resist family rules and boundaries. Teenagers can also become preoccupied with issues of justice and may wish to seek revenge on any third party involved in the parent's injuries (they may need support from outside the family in dealing with these strong emotions).

Some children, irrespective of their age, may not show outward signs of being affected and this can lead adults to assume that there are no problems. In some situations, children can even show improvement in their behaviour when faced with stressful situations; this may be the equivalent to an adult's attempts to 'keep busy' as a way of distracting themselves from their worries. These children may need support just as much as children who show their distress openly.

> Despite the child problems described here, it is important to note that most children are resilient when faced with crisis and are spared the more negative effects of this experience.

Ways of helping children

Giving children information and explaining head injury

Like adults, children need information to help them make sense of head injury and the issues and changes they have experienced as a result of it. It is particularly important to provide children with information because in its absence (especially if they are very young) they have a tendency to create their own explanation of events, which can often be inaccurate and more distressing than the 'truth'. Despite this, children do not typically receive adequate information when a relative is injured. Why not?

- Adults (understandably) worry that children might be upset by discussion of their relative's injury and so (misguidedly) try to protect them from this. However, in our experience children *do* want information and report feeling less upset when they know what is happening.

- Head injury staff may feel that they do not have the expertise to discuss issues in a way that children will understand, and so they too avoid talking to them. They might also feel anxious about dealing with children's distress, or lack the confidence to advise parents on supporting children. To add to this there are few published sources of information about head injury written specifically for children.

As a result of this adults can find themselves struggling to know how best to help children cope.

How do you explain head injury to children?

It helps to start by knowing what children of different ages typically understand and misunderstand about head injury. Children's understanding of illness and injury (in general) tends to increase as they get older, with teenagers and young adults having quite a sophisticated view of illness, while younger children see it in much simpler terms. The same is thought of their understanding of head injury. As a result, it is helpful to provide information at a level that is suitable for your child to understand. Key issues for you to bear in mind are discussed below.

◆ **Babies and infants (up to the age of 2 years)** The concept of a head injury is largely incomprehensible but they are aware of simple concepts such as being 'hurt' and 'sick', so these terms can be used when telling them what has happened to the relative. From around the age of 6 months babies become more aware of (and distressed by) the absence of a parent (especially if it is the mother and the separation is prolonged). Even very young children are sensitive to the 'emotional atmosphere' in the family and will pick up on and sense distress in others.

◆ **Pre-schoolers (up to the age of 5 years)** As language and thinking become more developed pre-schoolers have a greater understanding of what an injury is. However, they are likely to struggle to understand some aspects of head injury, such as the more 'unseen' problems (e.g. poor concentration) and may not understand that the injured person has ongoing difficulties if they look well. They will also find the idea of problems being long term or permanent difficult to understand, and so they are likely to expect the relative to make a full recovery.

A very important issue to bear in mind with this age group is that they typically view everything in relation to themselves (called 'egocentric' thinking) and so are extremely vulnerable to blaming themselves for the accident. Very young children have told us that they believe their parent's accident happened because they (the child) had been 'naughty' that day. Children may not tell you about these beliefs without some encouragement, because they feel guilty and distressed. Therefore we have found that it is very important to reassure all, but especially younger, children that they are not to blame for the injury (whether or not they feel that they are).

Children of this age can also be afraid that they will 'catch' the injury from their relative and so may avoid them. They will also be likely to ask you to repeat information many times and frequently ask questions about what you have told them.

◆ **Young school age children (age 6–12 years)** Children in this age group are capable of having a more sophisticated understanding of head injury; for example, they will understand both its 'seen' aspects (such as physical problems) and its 'unseen' aspects (such as cognitive problems) if they are clearly explained. However, they are still likely to expect the injured person to make a full recovery, and so may need help in understanding the long-term nature of head injury. Children of this age can be very concerned about what their friends will think about their relative (as they do not like feeling different) and so will need help knowing what to tell peers. This can be a very difficult issue for these children and they can be vulnerable to teasing. They, too, may blame themselves for their relative's injuries and may try to compensate for this by trying to help them recover—this may be through the belief that they must not misbehave and so they may become overly helpful at home. If so, they may need help in knowing how to behave 'normally' towards the relative.

- **Older school age children and teenagers** Young people in this age group can generally comprehend the complexity of head injury (in much the same ways as adults), and so can be told about issues such as the severity, seriousness, extent of recovery, and permanence of the injury. However, they will need considerable emotional support to be able to cope with this information.

Before giving your children information, try to ascertain what they already understand about the injury (and what they would like to know). This will help you know where to begin and how to structure information.

Try to prepare what you are going to say in advance of talking to them. Taking into account their age and what they already know), follow the structure below:

- State what a head injury is (the information provided for children in Appendices 2 and 3 may be a good starting point).

- Say how the head injury specifically affects their relative (include all areas of difficulty).

- Reassure the child that the head injury is not contagious and they are not to blame for it.

- Focus on the injured person's strengths and abilities, so that a balanced picture is given.

- Discuss recovery and the likelihood of some long-term problems. Balance this with an optimistic statement about the future and reassure the child that the relative will still be involved with them. For example, you could tell a 4-year-old that 'Daddy cannot walk at the moment because his legs are not working after the accident. He is learning to use his wheelchair and when he gets really good at driving it he will be able to take you on his lap to the park in it.'

- Acknowledge that the child may be feeling sadness and fear, that this is normal, and that it will improve.

- Ask the child to repeat what you have said (so you can check for any misunderstandings).

- Ask the child if they have questions.

It is important to be prepared for some direct and difficult questions that could distress you (e.g. 'Will he ever walk again?'). It is usually best to give an honest answer where possible, although this can be upsetting for all involved. Very young children benefit from lots of physical contact (e.g. sitting on your lap) when being given 'bad' news. It is also important to see information giving as an ongoing process so that your children are constantly 'up to date' with what is going on.

> Most important of all is to remind yourself that there is not one 'correct' thing to tell children or a 'right' way to say it. A willingness to talk to them and to listen to their concerns is much more important than what is actually said.

What else can help children?

As well as being provided with information about head injury, there are a number of other ways that children can be supported.

Practical strategies

- Try to keep children's daily routines as 'normal' as possible (which can be very difficult in the early stages of the head injury). It helps if they can continue with after-school activities, clubs, and hobbies, but you may need to have extra help to maintain this.

- It is helpful not to have too many different people looking after your children (especially if they are babies or very young) as this can make them feel insecure.

- It is also preferable for them to be cared for in their own home (if possible) rather than going off to relatives.

- Tell the school what is happening—they may be able to offer some extra support and will be sympathetic if the children seem upset or show changes in their behaviour.

- Get advice on any extra help or benefits you could access (e.g. extra nursery sessions—your health visitor can often organize this to help you out).

Emotional support

- Most children cope well with regular information about what is happening to their relative combined with the chance to talk through their feelings with an adult they know and trust. They can often have many conflicting feelings towards the injured parent which they should be encouraged to discuss (e.g. they feel sorry for them but also resent all the changes that have occurred since the injury). They may also be afraid that they will have to undertake care tasks for the relative (e.g. take them to the toilet) and should be reassured that this will not be expected of them. Younger children might prefer to draw or 'play out' how they are feeling (using dolls, toy hospitals) rather than talk.

◆ If the relative is away from the family for a prolonged period (e.g. for inpatient rehabilitation), children need help to cope with this separation. Encourage regular visits to the relative (if practical) alongside telephone calls, e-mails, and letters. If visits are not possible it is helpful for the children to see photographs of the relative as they are, especially if they have changed significantly as a result of the injury. Children can be given a 'symbol' of the relative to have close, e.g. parent's sweater to cuddle or their perfume.

◆ If children are able to visit the rehabilitation unit, ask if they can observe and participate in their relative's therapy sessions. This provides an opportunity for children to spend time with their relative and to learn about head injury and its treatment. However, it is important to plan visits involving children carefully, and to avoid visiting when children are tired, which the injured person might find hard to tolerate.

◆ Encourage physical contact between the relative and children, although there may be some anxiety about this if the injured person has severe physical limitations.

◆ Children may need to relearn ways of communicating with relatives who have speech and language problems.

◆ Some children may need specialist support (e.g. if they are continually sad, their school work deteriorates significantly, or they are engage in risky behaviours such as drug/alcohol use). You should seek advice from your GP in the first instance or your relative's head injury team (if appropriate). Headway may also be able to offer family support. Children who had problems (with behaviour, learning, or family relationships) before the injury are at greater risk for having increased problems afterwards and so may need a 'closer eye' keeping on them.

◆ Children are best supported by adults who are managing their own stress. Therefore it is important to look after yourself in order to be able to look after others.

When do children need support?

Children need support and information throughout the whole of their relative's recovery, but there are key times when they might experience heightened levels of stress and may benefit from additional help.

Acute stages

Children may need:

◆ help to deal with the emotional shock of the accident

◆ honest answers about whether their relative might die

◆ information about ITU/medical equipment and machinery in advance of seeing the relative for the first time so that they are prepared.

Post-acute stage

Children may need:

- help in managing ongoing separation from the relative
- support in coping with changes in the relative
- clear explanations about what will happen to their relative after they leave hospital and why (e.g. move to rehabilitation)
- help in setting realistic expectations for the future
- help in coping with setbacks (e.g. if their relative does not make progress)
- help in understanding why the relative may not return home (e.g. due to behavioural problems)
- considerable ongoing emotional support in the event of the relative remaining in a reduced awareness state, PVS, or coma.

When the injured person's rehabilitation is finished/is discharged home

Children may need:

- help in preparing for the relative's return home (especially if they have changed significantly); it is not uncommon for children to resent the parent returning home, especially if the separation has been prolonged and new routines have been established.
- support so that they do not to take on the role of a carer.

Longer term

Children may need:

- ongoing emotional support to cope with the effects of living with someone with head injury
- help to make normal transitions, such as going to university and leaving home, which many children who have parents with chronic conditions find difficult because of guilt and worry that the family may not cope without their help
- help to cope with other stressful life events that can occur because of head injury (e.g. parents' divorce, house moves); this 'pile-up' of stress can be challenging for all the family.

Is it all bad for children who have head-injured relatives?

So far we have focused on the possible negative effects of family head injury on children; however, this is likely to be only one part of the picture. Research is beginning to show that coping with difficult situations can bring out the best in children and can have a positive effect on their overall development. When they are well supported through stressful experiences, some children say that it made them more emotionally mature, taught them important coping skills that they might not have otherwise learnt, and helped them see themselves as strong people. They also said that their relative's injury provided them with a different perspective on what was important in life and that they appreciated their family more after it.

❓ Frequently asked questions:

◆ **My children have not asked any questions about the accident so I haven't discussed it with them. Wouldn't it just upset them?**

It is usually best to discuss important family issues as openly and honestly as possible. It is possible that your children do not have any questions, although this is not common. It may be that they are trying to protect you by not raising the issue; perhaps they have sensed your distress about events and do not want to cause further upset. If information is given sensitively and suited to the child's age it should not cause stress. Not knowing the facts can be more distressing.

◆ **I have three children. Two of them seem to have coped well with my wife's head injury, but one of them is really struggling. Why is this? Have I done something wrong?**

No, this commonly occurs in families and does not mean that you have done anything wrong in supporting this child. As we said earlier, some family members will react differently from others to events—and there are often reasons for this. Ask yourself, was this child particularly close to the parent and so may have had a stronger reaction to the injury? Is this child dealing with any other problems at the moment or were they having difficulties before the injury? How old is this child? Did they understand the information they have been given about what has happened? Are the types of problems they are having 'typical' for their age (e.g. teenagers often experience emotional turmoil—this might not be related to the injury).

◆ **My partner used to do all the childcare, but since his head injury I'm not sure he is safe to be left with the children. How can I tackle this?**

Someone's safety to parent after head injury is a very important but sensitive topic and, surprisingly, not one that is addressed by many rehabilitation services. You have raised an important issue, so try to enlist the help of any professionals working with your partner so that they can advise. Ask your GP or health visitor if there is a special parenting service in your area that you could be referred to (often provided by children's mental health services). If you are concerned about the safety of any child, it is important to seek help and advice from your GP, local Social Services Department (see the telephone book for your local office), or the NSPCC.

11

The longer term

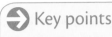
As you will have seen throughout this book, it is very difficult to make an accurate prediction of recovery and progress after a head injury. The effects of head injury on the family can be lifelong, requiring the family to make considerable adjustments to many aspects of their lives.

Every head injury is unique and each individual and their family will have a different experience, taking different pathways through the head injury journey. As you have seen from earlier chapters, spontaneous changes to the brain occur in the months and even first years after injury. This period of recovery continues for much longer than initially thought, but does slow down over time and usually leaves some longer-term difficulties.

While a negative outcome is not inevitable, if your relative does have persisting problems in the areas described (particularly in behaviour and thinking) it can be very hard to get back to normal family and work life. In many instances it is not possible to resume life as it was before, or fully resume previous roles and interests. The individual with the injury and the family are then faced with adjusting to changes in lifestyle, family roles, ways of being together, financial circumstances, and a future that may seem uncertain. As outlined earlier, this process of adjustment takes time and differs for everyone. There are key practical issues faced by families in the longer-term. Returning to driving and work are often primary long-term goals but return rates after head injury are disappointing. These two issues, together with the financial and legal aspects of head injury, are discussed below.

Returning to work after head injury

Return to employment is usually a major goal. Apart from the financial security that working can bring, it also gives us a sense of purpose and identity, enhances our self-esteem and confidence, and gives our time a sense of structure. Individuals can often feel a real sense of loss when they suddenly have to stop working.

Returning to work after a head injury can be challenging, even if the initial head injury was mild and the ongoing effects quite subtle. While most people return to work after a mild injury, this is less likely after a moderate or severe injury. Research and clinical evidence suggests that only about a third of people with more severe injuries return to work following head injury.

What makes return to work difficult?

Resuming work after head injury may be problematic for a number of reasons, for example:

♦ There may be issues related to the nature and severity of the head injury itself. Getting back to work can be very difficult if the injured person has ongoing difficulties such as physical, cognitive, communication, fatigue, or behavioural problems. They may not be ready for work if these problems are significant; in particular a return to work is likely to be unsuccessful if your relative is still trying to manage emotional problems, has difficulties interacting with others, or has reduced insight into their problems.

♦ There may also be factors related to the job itself. Important issues that can all have a significant impact on the individual's chances of returning successfully are:

  ♦ the complexity of the job (it is likely to be more difficult to return to a role such as an air traffic controller or surgeon after head injury than to a post of sales assistant because of the risks attached to the former)

  ♦ the availability of the job (Is your relative's old job being held open?)

  ♦ the hours required to complete the post (Could your relative manage full-time work?)

  ♦ the supportiveness of the employer

  ♦ the suitability of the work environment (Can it be adapted to take your relative's wheelchair? Is there a lot of background noise?)

  ♦ the travelling distance to the place of work.

Planning return to work

If your relative is thinking of returning to work it is important to ensure that their chances of doing this successfully are maximized. It can be extremely demoralizing for all involved if this is not properly thought through and goes wrong.

What can help?

♦ **Discuss with your relative (and any therapists involved in their care, such as occupational therapists and clinical psychologists) their view of their readiness to return to work** Are they aware of their problems and how these could impact on the work role? Discussion of the results of any formal assessments that have been undertaken (e.g. neuropsychological assessments (of memory and concentration) and workplace assessments) may be helpful. Are they motivated to address these problems before attempting a gradual resumption of formal work? It is not unusual for some individuals to return to work without any support because they are not anticipating any problems at all. Difficulties at work may then occur and seem to come out of the blue. This can be the first time the injured person realizes that their head injury is causing them problems and it may also be the first time that they seek help or that it is offered. Therefore it is important that the injured person, the employer, and those supporting the process begin from a realistic starting point.

♦ **Carefully plan a gradual and slow return to work** This will involve thinking carefully about each of the factors listed above and deciding how issues will be addressed. A key issue is being clear about what job the injured person is planning to return to—many people resume working for their old company but not necessarily in their previous role. It can be difficult for some injured people to consider taking on a 'lesser' duty. A graded approach to returning to work might involve initially only working for a few hours a week, which are gradually increased as the person's levels of stamina and tolerance develop. Many head-injured people want to resume work as quickly as possible and may be unwilling to follow this step-by-step approach, and they require family support and encouragement to do so. You can also help your relative by working with them on developing their use of any recommended compensatory aids and strategies, such as diaries and reminder systems, so that they can use these efficiently and effectively in the workplace. In addition, your relative might consider having a 'mentor' (or trusted colleague) at work who can give honest feedback about how the return is going. This type of feedback can be invaluable.

♦ **Seek as much help and as many resources as possible to support your relative's return to work** Specialist support may be offered by a range of professionals such as occupational therapists, clinical psychologists, disability employment advisors (based at your local Job Centre (part of the Jobcentre Plus service)), and charitable organizations such as Rehab UK. Headway may be able to tell you if a specialist vocational rehabilitation team exists in your area. The occupational health service at your relative's place of work can also be a useful starting point. These professionals may offer advice, help identify trial work placements, and offer ongoing work-place support. Help from rehabilitation teams and vocational rehabilitation services can make a big difference.

◆ **Be realistic about the effect of returning to work on the rest of the family** Contrary to many people's expectation that normal life will be resumed once the injured person gets back to work, family life can actually become more stressful. It is not unusual for families to see an increase in their relative's levels of fatigue and irritability at home as they put all their effort into 'holding things together' at work. This should gradually improve over time, but if not this could be an indicator that the process of returning to work needs to be more gradual.

What if your relative's return to work is unsuccessful?

For many people, return to their previous work is not a realistic option and they may need considerable support with the difficult issue of what to do instead. There may be a number of alternatives. Could doing voluntary work help them get back into a work role? If so, it may be helpful to seek advice from an occupational therapist in setting this up. Could your relative try to seek employment elsewhere? This opens up the issue of completing application forms and being interviewed, all of which can be more challenging for people to undertake after injury or illness. As a result, they may need support to do this.

Some people may never be able to resume work, which can be distressing for them and their families. In such cases emotional support and counselling may be necessary. After a period of adjustment they may be willing to consider developing their leisure time and finding other ways of structuring their time. This can be especially challenging for those who were still in education or training or just establishing themselves in their chosen career when they were injured. However, it is a really important factor in helping the injured person regain self-esteem.

Leisure activities

Leisure and hobbies are an important part of many people's lives. In similar ways to work, occupying our time meaningfully and enjoyably gives us pleasure, contributes to our self-identity, and can enhance our physical and emotional health. For many people, taking part in leisure pursuits can be their main means of being in contact with others. Unfortunately, head injury can significantly impact on a person's ability to participate in many leisure activities.

Physical difficulties may be the primary problem for many injured people, especially for sports and outdoor activities. Some of these problems can be compensated for in some hobbies. For example, a wide range of adaptive devices are available that can enable people with physical impairments to continue gardening from their wheelchair. Similarly, many wheelchair users participate in sports such as basketball. Information on adaptive devices and equipment can be obtained from your local occupational therapy service or via Dialability (a national service providing information and advice on specialist equipment and aids).

Ongoing cognitive problems can be also a major barrier to resuming many hobbies, affecting everyday 'taken for granted' activities such as doing the crossword, completing a jigsaw, or taking part in the local pub quiz. Reduced concentration, problems with remembering, or difficulties with speech can all impact on the injured person's ability to take part in such activities. This can also have an impact on the rest of the family, especially if these were activities that were enjoyed together. In many cases things can be done to compensate (see Chapter 5 for advice on managing problems with thinking skills) such as taking regular breaks and managing fatigue and background noise. However, in some instances it might be difficult to compensate for problems (e.g. a pub will nearly always be noisy and your relative may not be able to cope with this level of distraction).

Being unable to resume previously enjoyed activities can contribute to low mood for many people, especially if this is coupled with having to make adjustments in other aspects of their life, such as work or driving. Specialist advice on ways to return to old activities (and to pursue new ones) can be sought from some occupational therapy services. Headway and other day services in your area may also be able to support you and your relative with this. This may need to be undertaken in conjunction with supportive counselling for your relative if they need more formal help in coming to terms with the changes.

The loss of the injured person's leisure interests can be difficult for families to cope with as well. Aside from having to deal with your relative's distress, you are likely to have to adjust to having your relative with you for longer periods of time. This might seriously impact on your own social and leisure time, especially if your relative is not safe to be left alone. You may also find yourself having to participate in your relative's hobbies and interests more than previously (or more than you would like!) because of the level of support that they need to carry these out. This needs to be carefully negotiated with your relative so that arguments are prevented and expectations are clear. It might help to seek a volunteer to support your relative with their leisure interests—this could be a willing friend. They will need clear and honest information about your relative (e.g. if there is the chance that they could be incontinent on a trip out, say so, so that they are prepared for this). You might also want to consider contacting a local 'befriending' scheme (such as the Ryder–Cheshire Association) who can link your relative with a volunteer who will support them in their leisure activities. This can also provide families with much needed time alone. Your local branch of Headway might also provide day services where people with head injury can meet others and enjoy organized leisure activities and day trips out.

If you are researching leisure activities yourself via the Internet, your local county council website can also be a good starting point.

Medical advice should be sought on whether it is safe to resume sports and hobbies that may be regarded as potentially dangerous, such as contact sports (e.g. rugby and boxing) or some outdoor pursuits (e.g. rock climbing). Advice offered to your relative on when and how to return to previous sporting activities will depend not only on the nature of the head injury and whether your relative has developed epilepsy, but also on the sport and the level to which your relative is hoping to return.

Many people will return to sport after head injury, physical restrictions permitting, without concern. However, if you or a relative has been competing at a professional level before a head injury there may be specific guidelines or rules to consult before rushing back in at a pre-head injury pace. Examples where guidance is clear include boxing and rugby. At the professional sports level, additional checks will need to be made with insurance agencies and others. Whatever the level and form of sport your relative is planning to return to, it is usually advisable to return in a graded way to avoid incurring new injuries and to prevent fatigue.

Travelling and holidays form a significant part of leisure for many people, but there may be practical concerns and worries about a person's safety to travel after head injury. Whether and when your relative is safe to fly after their head injury will depend on so many factors that it would be misleading to offer advice other than to discuss this with the doctors who know your relative and with any travel insurance company or airline you are planning to use. If your relative has had any surgery, you may wish to make sure that there are no specific time restrictions associated with the surgical condition. Practical problems when travelling (e.g. access issues, travelling with a wheelchair) can be tackled with advance planning and some research into any help that might be available to you from airlines and other carriers. Take advantage of the opportunity to board flights ahead of other passengers and accept any assistance offered. Dialability can offer advice on accessible hotels and holiday accommodation as well as travel insurance for people with long-term health problems.

Driving

Driving is of great importance to many people in modern life, especially if they live in rural or isolated areas. Driving often gives us a real sense of independence and control. Therefore being unable to drive after head injury can lead to a number of practical problems and be another source of stress.

Although some people will be able to return to driving as soon as they are fully recovered, for others it is not possible (e.g. if they have had surgery to their brain or have had one or more epileptic seizures, or if they are at high risk of having one since the head injury).

Driving is a highly complex skill, which draws on many different functions. First, there are the physical aspects of driving. In order to drive, an individual needs to be able to manipulate the gear stick, reach the pedals, see adequately, and so on. Driving also requires a number of complex thinking skills, such as attention (e.g. being able to stay focused on driving and ignore distractions), speed of information processing (e.g. being able to respond quickly to someone stepping into the road unexpectedly), memory (e.g. remembering your route), being able to make quick decisions, and visual perception (in order to make sense of the visual information coming in from all around). Over time, after we learn to drive, driving becomes an automatic skill that we rarely think about—if you think back to when you were first learning to drive you may remember how difficult (and tiring!) it was to draw on all these skills when they were not so automatic.

For everyone's safety there are very clear rules about driving after a head injury. It is illegal to drive if you are unfit to do so (and you will not be covered by your insurance policy if you do drive). Therefore after a head injury your relative has a legal responsibility to inform the Driving Vehicle License Association (DVLA) and their insurance company about the injury. If they are unable to do this, someone else within the family will need to take responsibility for contacting these organizations. The details of the DVLA are provided in Appendix 1. They will send a form for your relative or you to complete, and may contact your relative's doctor for information. In some cases, they may arrange an independent assessment.

The information used by the DVLA to advise head-injured people when it is safe to resume driving is constantly being updated. Your doctor can give you more information about this. At the time of writing (January 2008), the advice is as follows.

- If there has been full physical, visual, and cognitive recovery after a brain injury, someone who had a single seizure in the first 24 hours after their brain injury may be permitted to return to driving within 12 months as long as they have not had further seizures.

- Also, if someone has seizures but they have only occurred at night for over 3 years, the DVLA may advise that it is safe to resume driving.

- There are also considerations to be made if, after returning to drive, any medication for seizures is being changed. If an anticonvulsant is being discontinued, the driver is obliged to inform the DVLA. The DVLA usually requests a letter from the doctor advising on the change in treatment and often advise that driving is ceased for 6 months. The reason for this is that there is a risk of seizures recurring when anticonvulsant medication is stopped, even if there have been no fits for many years.

If your relative has had brain surgery, there will be a minimum 6 months ban from driving. The DVLA will then decide whether he/she can start driving again. They usually do this on the basis of information collected from doctors and other professionals involved in your relative's care. In some cases, your relative may be referred for an independent driving assessment before he/she is able to drive again. There are many specialist centres around the country that offer this service. They can also give advice on car adaptations if needed, and offer driving and refresher lessons.

> **Remember** The information used by the DVLA to advise head-injured people when it is safe to resume driving is constantly being updated. Contact the DVLA directly or your doctor for more information. It is also important to seek advice if you are learning to drive (i.e. you have a provisional license) or are considering learning after a head injury.

Finances

Your family income can be significantly affected after a head injury. This may only be on a short-term basis (e.g. in the stages of initial recovery after mild head injury) but is typically a longer-term problem facing most families. This might be because your relative is not working (at least in the initial stages of recovery) or is unable to return to work in the long term, or because you and other family members are unable to work (or can only work in a reduced capacity) because of your commitments to caring for your relative.

There are a wide range of benefits to which your relative may be entitled. Whether your relative is entitled to any will depend very much on their individual circumstances. The Citizen's Advice Bureau in the UK is one of the best sources of information and support with all of the above. There are also some useful leaflets and websites (e.g. the Department of Work and Pensions website (www.dwp.gov.uk) provides an overview of the benefits system). The completion of benefits application forms can be complex, especially when an injured person's primary problems are not physical (these can usually be ticked off in boxes much more easily than cognitive problems); therefore it is advisable to have help from someone experienced in this when you are completing your applications. Again, Headway (staff or other families) may be an invaluable source of information and support. Similarly, you should seek advice on how to appeal if you are refused a benefit that you believe you are entitled to.

This issue of finances leads us to another important issue—whether your relative is able to manage and deal with financial and other complex issues after their injury.

Legal issues
Obtaining legal representation after a head injury

Legal issues surrounding head injury can be very complex. The context in which a head injury may occur is diverse: road traffic accidents, sporting accidents,

accidents at work, and medical or clinical negligence to mention just a few. As stated elsewhere in this book, the head injury may be invisible to others. Therefore it is important to find a legal representative who is fully aware that head injury may cause physical, cognitive, and emotional problems.

There are a number of law firms who specialize in the field of head injury. It is advisable for somebody seeking legal advice following a head injury to find a legal representative who has experience in handling such cases. Often the best way of locating the right solicitor is through the advice of healthcare professionals who may be knowledgeable of which solicitors regularly handle head injury claims. Headway can also provide a list of personal injury solicitors who specialize in head injury. Of course there are numerous firms advertising personal injury law and associations for law firms specializing in personal injury on the Internet. The key is to locate a firm that specializes in head injury cases.

A head injury can significantly change the lives of the person and their family. Claiming compensation is one way of trying to achieve some stability and support in order to improve or maintain independence and quality of life.

Frequently asked questions about compensation claims

* **How much time do I have to make my claim?**

   The general rule is 3 years from the date of the accident, but there are exceptions that your legal representative can give advice on.

* **How much compensation is paid out to somebody with a head injury?**

   There is no standard amount of compensation for any particular type of injury. Each case is assessed individually on its merits.

* **What is an interim payment?**

   An interim payment is an amount paid in partial settlement of a claim. Sometimes somebody with a severe head injury needs private rehabilitation costs or their accommodation adapted for them. Such a payment(s) would be made to facilitate recovery whilst consideration is given to the award for the full amount of losses.

* **How much will I have to pay the solicitor?**

   Most specialist reputable firms recover legal fees from the person responsible for the individual's head injury or their insurers. In criminal cases where somebody has been assaulted and sustained a head injury the claim is dealt with by the Criminal Injuries Compensation Authority (CICA).

The medico-legal assessment process

Central to the legal process is obtaining information as to the effect of the head injury on the individual concerned. Specialist reports may be obtained from a number of clinicians including medical consultants, clinical neuropsychologists, occupational and other therapists (e.g. speech and language therapists, physiotherapists), and nursing and care experts. Often the solicitors for both the claimants and the defendants (or the defendants' insurers) instruct their own experts so the person who has the head injury will have to attend a number of examinations as part of his/her medico-legal claim. This can be a time-consuming and stressful process.

Individuals who sustain head injury often do not have good insight into the nature of their problems. This phenomenon is sometimes related to the nature of the injury to the frontal lobes of the brain and/or that the patient is denying aspects of his/her condition. The most accurate description of how somebody's behaviour has changed following a head injury typically comes from close relatives or friends. Therefore it is common for specialists involved in the medico-legal process to want to ask questions of family members. Indeed, in addition to this, solicitors will often take witness statements from family members regarding the changes observed in their clients post-injury.

Stress associated with the medico-legal process

Head injury compensation claims will frequently raise complex issues. In the aftermath of a critical life event individuals and their families are frequently coping with the immediate physical, psychological, and emotional consequences of the head injury. They are not necessarily focused on future planning and any associated legal issues. Indeed, such considerations may appear somewhat out of kilter with what has happened as individuals are trying to adjust to a traumatic life event. However, accessing practical advice and support in relation to legal issues can help to clarify questions regarding what has happened and what can be done to help.

It is important to realize that compensation claims are rarely settled speedily. The medico-legal process itself can be particularly stressful for the individual sufferer and his/her family, carers, and friends. Therefore it is advisable, where at all possible, to be open with professionals, including solicitors, doctors, and other clinicians about the stresses involved so that advice and support is made available where possible. Indeed, experienced solicitors will frequently try to access specialist counselling support for their clients and family members as part of the claims process.

Legislation to protect individuals who lack capacity to make specific decisions for themselves

Issues regarding an individual's ability to make decisions can arise following head injury for the reasons outlined in this book. The effect of the head injury may range from mild problems with attention, concentration, and memory to the severely injured who remain in a comatose or persistent vegetative condition. There is new legislation in the UK to protect people who cannot make decisions for themselves, including those who have suffered head injury. **The Mental Capacity Act 2005** came fully into force on 1 October 2007. It provides clear guidelines for carers and professionals about who can take decisions in which situations.

The Mental Capacity Act clearly states that everybody over 16 should be treated as able to make decisions until it is shown otherwise. The Act also aims to enable people to make their own decisions for as long as they are capable of doing so. Furthermore, the law recognizes the right of individuals to make unwise decisions. The Mental Capacity Act states that:

An adult can only be considered unable to make a particular decision if:

1. he or she has an impairment of, or disturbance in, the functioning of the mind or brain, whether permanent or temporary,

    AND

2. he or she is unable to take any of the following steps:

    - understand the information relevant to the decision
    - retain that information
    - use or weigh that information as part of the decision-making process
    - communicate the decision made (whether by talking, sign language, or other means.

When assessing somebody's ability to make a decision, the assessor must follow the above steps.

When assessing someone's capacity to make a decision we have to state very clearly what decision we are referring to. This is because it is possible for someone to be able to make decisions competently about one aspect of their life (e.g. whether to have a medical treatment or not) but not have the capacity to make a decision about another area of their life (e.g. how to handle their money) because they have cognitive problems.

When someone lacks capacity regarding a decision

The Act intends to protect people who lose the capacity to make their own decisions. It will:

- Allow the person, while they are still able, to appoint someone (for example a trusted relative or friend) to make decisions on their behalf once they lose the ability to do so. This will mean that person can make decisions on the person's health and personal welfare. In the past the law only covered financial issues.

- Ensure that decisions that are made on the person's behalf are in their best interests.

- The Act provides a checklist of things that decision makers must work through.

People with no one to act for them will also be able to leave instructions for their care under the new provisions.

Independent Mental Capacity Advocate

The Mental Capacity Act set up a new service, the Independent Mental Capacity Advocate (IMCA) service. The service will help vulnerable people who cannot make some or all important decisions about their lives.

The IMCA service will mean that certain people who lack capacity, including people with head injury, will be helped to make difficult decisions such as medical treatment choices or where they would like to live. It is aimed at people who lack family or friends to speak for them.

The Office of the Public Guardian

The Office of the Public Guardian (OPG) protects people who lack the mental capacity to make decisions for themselves. It does this through regulating and supervising court-appointed deputies, and by registering Lasting Powers of Attorney (LPAs) and Enduring Powers of Attorney (EPAs).

Lasting Powers of Attorney

An attorney is someone who can advise on legal matters and represent you in court. Lasting Powers of Attorney replace Enduring Powers of Attorney. LPAs will give vulnerable people greater choice and control over their future and enable people to choose someone they trust to look after their affairs if necessary.

LPAs cover personal welfare as well as finance and property decisions. As they can only be used after they have been registered with the Public Guardian, they will be under more scrutiny and ensure that any decisions made on behalf of people lacking capacity are in their best interests.

In some cases, where there are suspicions that an attorney or deputy might not be acting in the best interests of the person they represent, the OPG will work with other organizations to investigate any allegations of abuse. There is a new criminal offence of neglect or ill-treatment of a person who lacks capacity.

The OPG also provides information on mental capacity to the public and can provide contacts with other organizations working in the field of mental capacity.

The Court of Protection

The Court of Protection deals with all issues relating to people who lack the capacity to make specific decisions regarding, for example, financial or serious health care matters. It will look at cases where there is disagreement on what the person's best interests are. The Court of Protection has specially trained judges to deal with decisions relating to personal welfare, as well as property and financial affairs.

What has been outlined above with regard to the Mental Capacity Act frequently raises more questions and potential anxiety. Rather than individuals and their families becoming anxious and wading through policy documents about such issues, it makes sense to access professionals and agencies such as Headway who are more familiar, and resourced, to offer advice and education on such topics. The Act itself has as its central purpose the protection and best interests of vulnerable adults. Issues relating to capacity do not always arise following head injury. However, when they do, collaboration between the injured party, family and carers, clinicians, and legal representatives will better ensure that the individual's best interests are indeed met.

Longer-term family adjustment: learning to live with head injury in the family

Throughout this book we have stressed that head injury typically requires lifelong adjustment for the injured person and their families. In the early stages of recovery, this process is driven by the desire to 'get back to normal'. However, as time passes, families gradually experience a growing realization that the old way of life has changed permanently for all of them and a new sense of 'normal' has to be achieved. What follows is usually an ongoing rearrangement and readjustment of family routines, duties, roles, expectations, and values. Ultimately this can lead to a sense of the head injury becoming integrated within family life. However, it is fair to say that there is typically no 'endpoint' to this process (families rarely say that they have 'accepted' the injury, as this notion is often associated with 'giving in') and many years on most people are still 'learning to live with it'. As you will have read earlier, for many families this can be a positive process, in which a range of new strengths and values are discovered and family relationships and bonds are strengthened.

What helps families cope in the long term?

The following can help to support other family members and family life.

- ◆ **Continue to review family roles and responsibilities** Things will gradually change over time (for better *and* for worse, and often without you noticing) and it can help to 'take stock' every now and again. Perhaps review how duties are shared and ask whether any alterations are required in order to accommodate other (non head injury-related) family changes. For example, you may have been your relative's primary carer but now wish to resume work. To whom and how will your duties be reassigned? Do your children need a period of time when they are able to help less with the injured person because they are due to take school examinations? Is everyone in the family happy with the allocation of duties, and if not, how can difficulties be addressed? Regular family meetings can help avoid the build-up of unspoken stress and concerns.

◆ **Try not to view your entire world through the lens of the head injury** Not all the challenges you will face in the coming years (e.g. difficult teenagers, financial concerns) will be as a direct result of the head injury (although inevitably some will be). Thinking through the source of any problems will help you identify the best course of action and the best options for support.

◆ **Try, as far as you feel able, to re-establish some of your old family routines and activities** After head injury, there can be a tendency to discontinue family traditions (such as the whole family meeting for the annual summer barbecue) because of a belief that life can never be the same again, or that it is wrong to have fun when your injured relative is still experiencing difficulties or is not living with the family. Research has shown that families that resume a 'normal' family life, as far as they are able, as well as maintaining their sense of humour generally fare better in the long term. This is not always easy and will take time. It is especially important to try to achieve this if you still have young children living with you.

Research tells us that families' support networks diminish in the longer term, especially as services withdraw (usually at a time when they are needed most). Therefore it is important to try to establish (or re-establish) a strong social support network, comprising family, friends, and services. Do not be afraid of asking for more support, even if it is many years since the initial injury occurred.

In the longer term, many families will be continuing to deal with the persisting effects of the head injury. It helps to continue to use the strategies that you have already found helpful and to seek specialist advice and support from services if you feel that you are no longer coping with previously well-managed problems. This is particularly relevant for families whose relative continues to show behavioural problems, as we know from research that this problem causes families the greatest long-term stress. You may also wish to seek information on more practical forms of support including day care for your relative or respite (a place where your relative may go and stay for short periods of time) so that you and the rest of the family have a break from your caring responsibilities. Some families are not able to cope with severe and ongoing behavioural problems in the long term and will request that their relative is accommodated elsewhere. This can be a very difficult decision to reach, and local head injury teams and social services care managers can support families facing such situations. Family counselling alongside this can also help. Such decisions may also be accompanied by other major and potentially stressful life events, such as moving house or divorcing the injured person. Children in families facing these situations require considerable support to manage the 'pile-up' of stress that can be experienced.

As well as supporting your injured relative, you are likely to need to go on supporting others in the family. This can be challenging and demanding, but children in particular need support and information that is ongoing, up to date, and relates directly to the current family circumstances. Research has shown that when children are given this kind of continued support and information about family illness they generally cope better.

Taking care of yourself and preventing 'burn out'

It is also important for you to have a 'blueprint' for coping in the future, particularly if you are your injured relative's main carer. The following might help:

- **Gain the support of your GP** Once your relative is no longer in touch with head injury services, your GP will be your first port of call, along with Headway, for advice and help. It is useful to try to establish a good collaborative working relationship with him/her and for you to ensure that he/she is familiar with your injured relative and his/her needs.

- **Make contact with your local branch of Headway** As you read this you may not feel that you will need their support, but if this changes over time it will be useful to have already familiarized yourself with what they can offer.

- **Pay attention to how you are feeling** It is important to **recognize the signs of burnout**. These include increased irritability, feeling overwhelmed, feeling unable to cope, severe fatigue and exhaustion, sleep problems, and possible feelings of guilt and resentment (to name a few). What to do:

  - seek advice from your GP
  - counselling might help—ask your GP or Headway about what is available
  - recognize your own limits
  - make time for yourself on a regular basis—and do pleasurable things (have a massage or a beauty treatment, play golf, or take a long walk)
  - pursue a hobby or attend a class
  - practice relaxation
  - try not to feel guilty when taking this time for yourself
  - tap into your support network and learn to ask for what you need
  - become comfortable with accepting help
  - join a carers support group.

On a positive note

While much of this book has focused on the problems and difficulties associated with head injury, it is important to end on a positive note for the picture is not totally bleak. The process of recovering from head injury (for both the injured person and their family), while challenging, is not always negative. Families often report positive changes, such as having more time together as a family, the strengthening of relationships, and having enhanced ability to cope with life stress.

Conclusions

You may be reading, or re-reading, this book at any stage of your relative's recovery from head injury. We hope whatever stage of this journey that you are at, you find something useful to take forward. As we have repeatedly stressed throughout this book your relative's head injury—and your family's experience of this—will be unique. On the one hand this means that it is not possible to get definite answers to all your questions or accurate predictions of what to expect next. We know that this level of uncertainty can be extremely hard to deal with. On the other hand, however, it may also leave you with a degree of hope. Families do adjust and deal with changes in their roles and relationships—and the key is finding out what works for you as a family and identifying the support that is available to you.

Appendix 1

Resources and further reading

General

Headway—the national brain injury association for the UK. The national contact will have a directory of local groups. 7 King Edward Court, King Edward Street, Nottingham, NG1 1EW. National Helpline number: 0808-8002244; www.headway.org.uk

BASIC—Brain and Spinal Injury Centre national helpline. Tel. 0800 750 0000

UKABIF UK Acquired Brain Injury Forum—directory of rehabilitation services for ABI within the UK (2005): www.ukabif.org.uk

www.rehabuk.org—Provides information on rehabilitation services throughout the UK (divided into geographical areas)

Carers UK 20–25 Glasshouse Yard, London, EC1A 4JT. Tel. 0808 8087777; www.carersuk.org

NHS Direct Health encyclopedia–head injury: www.nhsdirect.nhs.uk

www.braininjury.co.uk—Free site providing information and links about brain injury

Brain and Spine Foundation: www.brainandspine.org.uk

British Epilepsy Association—a national charity: www.epilepsy.org.uk

Brain Injury Rehabilitation Trust: www.birt.co.uk

National Service Framework for Long-term Conditions (2005): www.dh.gov.uk

Leonard Cheshire UK—charity provider of disability services: www.leonard-cheshire.org

Social services department for your area: listed in telephone directory

Citizen's Advice Bureau for your area: listed in telephone directory

Cognitive changes

Headway booklets: *Memory problems after brain injury* (B.Wilson); *Psychological effects of head injury* (A. Tyerman). Available from Headway.

Head injury: a practical guide by T. Powell (2004). Speechmark Publishing. Available from Headway.

Coping with memory problems: a practical guide for people with memory impairments, their relatives, friends and carers by L. Clare and B.A. Wilson (1997). Available from Harcourt Assessment (Tel. 01865 888188; www.harcourt-uk.com)

Internet resources: www.headway.org.uk; www.braininjury.com

Emotional and behavioural changes

Headway booklets: *Managing anger*; *Psychological effects of head injury*. Available from Headway.

Head injury: a practical guide by T. Powell (2004). Speechmark Publishing.

British Association for Counselling and Psychotherapy: lists accredited counsellors and psychologists within the UK. BACP house, 35–37 Albert Street, Rugby, CV1 2SG. Tel. 0870 4435252; www.babcp.org.uk

British Psychological Society: www.bps.org.uk

MIND 15–19 Broadway, London, E15 4BQ. Tel. 0845 7660163; www.mind.org.uk

Samaritans: 24-hour helpline. Tel. 0845 7909090; www.samaritans.org

Communication difficulties

Speakability—national and local support charity for people with aphasia. They produce useful information leaflets and advice. Royal Street, London SE1 7LL. Tel. 080 8808 9572 (helpline); www.speakability.org.uk

Connect—a charity for people with aphasia and their family and friends. They produce excellent publications, information, and courses for people with aphasia, their family and friends, and professionals: www.ukconnect.org

www.aphasiahelp.org: a website for people with aphasia

Royal College of Speech and Language Therapists: Tel. 020 7378 1200; www.rcslt.org

Sexual functioning
To find a relationship and psychosexual therapist

www.relate.org.uk (this also provides information about relationships, sexual problems, counselling on line, books about sex and relationships, and vibrators for women)

www.basrt.org.uk

www.pinktherapy.org.uk (therapy for people who are lesbian, gay, bisexual, and transgender)

For people wanting to meet others

www.outsiders.org.uk

www.disabilitynow.org.uk (general information including chat room and online dating)

www.icasa.co.uk (training organization that also provides sexual therapy and surrogate partners)

For information about sexual dysfunction, sexual health, and sexual aids

www.sda.uk.net (Sexual Dysfunction Association provides information about male and female sexual dysfunction)

www.bbc.co.uk/ouch (reflects the lives and experiences of people with disabilities; has regular columns, features, quizzes, and message boards)

www.bbc.co.uk/relationships (provides information about intimacy, conflict, sexual health, sexual problems, dating, and bereavement)

www.beecourse.com (supplies books informing about sexual health, relationships, and sexual problems; also supplies sexual aids and toys)

www.owenmumford.com (supplies sexual aids)

Supporting children

For adults

My Mum needs me by J. Segal and J. Simkins (1993) is actually about Multiple Sclerosis in the family but is a useful book for adults to read about children's reactions to parental illness generally

Lash Publishers (based in the USA) have an excellent range of publications for adults and children about head injury (and other disabilities). These can be ordered from their website: www.lapublishing.com

For children

The website www.kidshealth.org has a very useful section called "The brain is the boss" which teaches children how the brain works

My Mum/Dad has had a head injury is a booklet written for children by Wendy Murray, Social Worker, Lunan Park Resource Centre, Guthrie Street, Fr)ockheim, Arbroath, DD11 4SZ. Tel. 01241 826903. The booklet can be purchased directly from Ms Murray, but you could also ask your local head injury team if they have a copy

The Children's Brain Injury Trust (CBIT) has information leaflets about head injury for siblings: www.cbituk.org

Headway booklet: *My Dad's had a brain injury* (written for children). See their website (www.headway.org.uk) or ask your local Headway branch if they stock it (branch contact information can be found on their website)

There is an excellent Australian-based website for children (about the brain and injuries) at www.health.qld.gov.au. The children's section is called Brain Crew Kids Zone and contains 'Brain facts', 'Brain quizzes', and personal accounts of family head injury, written by children. The site also includes information for adults

Driving

Ricability (a charity publishing information on products and services for people with disabilities) 30 Angel Gate, City Road, London, EC1V 2PT. Tel. 020 7427 2460; www.ricability.org.uk. They also produce a booklet *Motoring after brain injury*

DVLA—Drivers Medical Unit, D6, DVLA, Longview Road, Swansea, SA99 1TU. Tel. 01792 783686

Headway booklet: *Driving after brain injury*

Driving after stroke (The Stroke Association)—although written for people who have had a stroke, this booklet provides useful information on car adaptations, and lists car modification firms and UK driving assessment centres

The Disabled Motorist (www.disabled-motorist.co.uk) produces information on all aspects of mobility and disability. Also produces a monthly magazine

Legal issues

Headway—provides excellent information, and care and support for people affected by brain injury. Tel. 0115 924 0800; www.headway.org.uk

Association of Personal Injury Lawyers: Tel. 0115 958 0585; www.apil.org.uk

Criminal Injuries Compensation Authority: Tel. 0800 358 3601; www.cica.gov.uk

Motor Insurance Bureau: Tel. 01908 830001; www.mib.org.uk

Mental Capacity Act 2005—information available at www.opsi.gov.uk/acts/acts2005

Independent Mental Capacity Advocate Service—information available at www.dh.gov.uk/socialcare

The Office of The Public Guardian and Court of Protection: Tel. 0845 3302900; www.publicguardian.co.uk

Some currently relevant published guidelines on the pathways, services, and treatments that should be available following head injury (March 2008)

National Service Framework (NSF) for Long-term Conditions (2005), Department of Health

This is often cited in public announcements from the UK Government and the Department of Health. It is not just about head injury but places emphasis on all long-term neurological conditions. It is perhaps worth mentioning that many of the recommendations cannot be carried out with the current level of staffing and resources in the UK National Health Service. The framework has been set up as a 10-year plan for gradual change. It is stated that the intention of this framework was that the services for all people would become more person and family centred, easier to access, and more equitable across the country. In addition, the pathways that patients and their families take through the various services are expected to become more stream lined, better coordinated, and easier to understand.

Medical rehabilitation for people with physical and complex disabilities: A report by The Royal College of Physicians Committee on Rehabilitation Medicine (2000)

This is much less high profile but it is used by rehabilitation professionals when auditing their own services or trying to develop them.

Head injury-specific guidelines

The following recent guidelines have been produced specifically on traumatic or acquired brain injury. They are produced to offer guidance to professionals working with head-injured people and their families, but cannot be used to specify what sort of treatment or support any particular person should be having at any particular time because every head-injured person will be in a very individual situation and professionals are expected to make their own judgements about what management and treatment is needed, depending on the exact nature of their patients situation.

Head injury—triage, assessment, investigation and early management of head injury in infants, children and adults. NICE (National Institute for Clinical Excellence), 2003 (updated 2007)

This includes excellent information produced for patients, carers, and families, and for the general public. It focuses on the early stages (first 48 hours) and includes guidance on what to do if someone has a head injury and what should happen in any admission to hospital and after discharge home. It does not discuss rehabilitation. These guidelines have recently been updated (2007).

Rehabilitation following acquired brain injury—national clinical guidelines. British Society of Rehabilitation Medicine and the Royal College of Physicians, 2003.

This complements the NICE guidelines and provides guidelines and sets standards of care and rehabilitation/treatment essential for the longer term to prevent the development of long-term complications and ensure that people return to as good a quality of life as possible following their injury.

International working party report on the vegetative state. The Royal Hospital for Neuro-disability, Putney, 1996.

This is still referred to by both medical and legal professionals. It is likely to be updated in the next few years.

Appendix 2

Information for younger children (aged 7–10)

This section should be read with a parent or an adult.

Brains, bones, and other body bits!

You are probably reading this because someone in your family (maybe your mum or dad) has had an injury. The injury they had is called a head injury.

When someone has a head injury it can be very upsetting and worrying for all the family, including you.

We hope that when you read this you will understand more about head injury. We can feel less afraid and worried when we know what is going on.

We also hope that it will help you to talk more to your family about what has happened. We can often feel more upset if we keep our feelings and worries inside.

We don't know how much you know already about the injury your relative had, but we are sure that you will have a few questions about it. You may read answers to some of your questions here. If you have any more questions, you could write them down and ask an adult to help you find the answer. There are also books and websites that can tell you more.

What is a head injury?

A head injury is when the head and the brain (which is inside the head) get hurt. Sometimes a head injury is called a brain injury. There is a drawing of the head and brain in Chapter 2.

Who can get a head injury?

Anyone can have a head injury. Men and women and girls and boys can have a head injury.

Why does a head injury happen?

Most people have a head injury because of an accident. This could be a car accident, falling off something high (like a ladder), or being hit on the head by something.

Many children we have spoken to were worried that they might have made their relative's injury happen—maybe because they had been naughty or by causing trouble.

Some children think they might have been able to stop the injury from happening or wish that they had been nicer to the person who got hurt.

It's normal to worry about this but, REMEMBER, your relative's injury did not happen because of anything you did and they would not want you to worry about this.

What happens when someone has a head injury?

Most people go to hospital when they have had a head injury. If their injury is very bad they might have to go in an ambulance or a special helicopter ambulance. This is scary for everyone (but a bit exciting too!). At the hospital their injury is looked at by doctors to see how bad it is and they are given tests (like X-rays) and sometimes medicine to stop them hurting.

After this, most people can go home and they usually get better quite soon. Some people, who have more serious injuries, will have to stay in hospital. This could be for months if they are very poorly. Everyone is different, and so it might take some people longer to start to feel better. They usually need help from different people at the hospital to get better. Children can usually go to visit their relative when they are in hospital and the staff might show you some things that you can do that you will both enjoy.

Most people do not die because of a head injury—but a few do. This is because the head injury was so bad that even the doctors could not make things better. This is very sad for everyone in the family and they need lots of help if this happens. You might have worried that your relative would die—lots of children feel like this—it helps to tell someone else in the family so they can talk to you about this and tell you what is happening.

What kinds of problems can people with head injuries have?

When someone has a head injury their brain is usually injured too. Hurting our brains can lead to many different types of problems. This is because the brain controls all of our body including our thinking, our talking, and how we feel and behave.

If you hurt one part of your brain, you will have one type of problem; if you hurt another part of the brain, you will have a different type of problem. This is because different parts of the brain all have different jobs. You could look at websites to learn more about the brain—it is fascinating.

People with head injuries may find it hard to control parts of their bodies. They might not be able to walk or use their arms as well as before. They may also have problems talking or understanding what people are saying (which can cause lots of upset and confusion), or they may find it hard to remember things or to concentrate. They may be more bad tempered or angrier than they used to be as well or perhaps very sad.

It can be very hard to understand the changes that head injury causes—the injured person can look exactly the same as they did before they were hurt but they can act differently. How they act can upset you, or make you angry or embarrassed. You might not want your friends to see them like this. Sometimes they can make you laugh too!

Try to remember that they have changed because of the accident—not because of anything you did and not because they want to upset you.

Do head injury problems get better?

Yes—lots of problems after a head injury can get better.

However, it can take a very long time for things to get better and even after many years people with head injuries can still have problems. It is very hard for the doctors to know who will get better and how long it will take—usually we just have to wait and see what happens.

Some people have problems that never go away, and this can make life hard for them and their families. Staff from the hospital will try to help families find new ways of doing things. Sometimes people with head injuries who have a lot of problems have to be looked after by people who are specially trained. This means that they have to live away from the family, which can be sad.

How does it feel to have a head injury?

We can't really know how it feels if we don't have the injury. People with head injures can be very upset about what has happened and worry about whether they will get better. They can seem sad or angry about it all. If people have problems with their memory, they might feel very confused and not know what is going on.

Other people who have head injuries are not as upset about it. Perhaps you could ask your relative how they are feeling—or ask another adult to tell you more.

How does the rest of the family feel when a head injury happens?

Every family gets upset and worried when someone has a head injury, especially as no one is sure what is going to happen.

The adults might be sad and crying; they might be at the hospital a lot and not have much time for you and your normal family things. This can make you feel annoyed. When the injured person comes home from hospital they might not be able to do the things they used to do, like drive the car or go to work, and other people in the family might have to take on some of their jobs. This can sometimes make people tired and upset. You might also have to do some extra jobs around the house to help out.

Sometimes the person with the head injury needs help to look after themselves, like having help to take a bath or to go to the toilet. If you are worried that you will have to help them do these things, talk to a grown-up.

There can be lots of changes to get used to after someone has a head injury—it can take time for things to feel OK again. It helps to tell someone when you are worried about anything.

How do children feel when head injury happens in the family?

Not everyone feels the same about head injury. Some children feel OK, but other children feel worried and sad and find it hard to get on with things. They don't enjoy school as much as before and might not do so well with their work. Also, they might not get on with others in the family as well as before. Many children have worries—about the person who is ill, about the rest of the family and about themselves. Feelings can get very mixed up. Some days they feel sad, and other days they might feel afraid. Some children are angry that the accident happened and feel that their life has been ruined. It is normal to feel like this for a while. The good thing is that these feelings don't last forever. It will help if you tell someone about them.

Remember, there is no right or wrong way to feel about a head injury; whatever you are feeling is OK.

What can help you feel better?

- Find out how the brain works and what can go wrong when it is injured. Children who have done this said it made them feel a bit better as they understood more.
- Try to remember that none of this was your fault.

- Talk to an adult whom you like and trust about your worries. They will help you find a way to feel better about things.
- It can help to write down your worries, questions, or feelings—perhaps in a special notebook.
- Try to remember that even though they have had an injury and may have changed, your relative still loves you.

Do you want to know more?

We hope that reading this has helped to answer some of the questions. However, there are always some questions that we haven't been able to answer you might have and we are sorry if we have missed yours out. It might help to speak to the adult who gave you this book. If you feel upset or worried, please talk to an adult straight away.

Ask your local library if they have any books about the brain. Also, here are some websites that you might want to look at:

- the website www.kidshealth.org has a great section called 'The brain is the boss' which teaches you how the brain works
- go to www.health.qld.gov.au and click on the children's section called Brain Crew Kids Zone which has fun 'Brain facts' and 'Brain quizzes'.

Appendix 3

Information for young people (aged 11–15)

Understanding head injury

This book is about head injury and you are probably reading this bit of it because someone in your family has been injured.

Head injury is a very common problem and many people are affected by it (see Chapter 2 of this book if you want to know more), so there will be many other young people, like you, dealing with this upsetting event.

Head injuries happen very suddenly, without warning, and so coping with them can be difficult. Therefore we have written this part of the book especially for you to try to help you through this experience. We hope it will help you to:

- **Understand more about head injury** Having information about something can help improve our understanding of it and possibly help us to feel less confused, worried and upset.

- **Find ways to get support and help for yourself** It can help to share your concerns and worries with someone you can trust. Difficult feelings can build up and become troublesome if kept to ourselves. However, talking to others about our feelings is not always easy, so we will also suggest other ways you can support yourself.

We don't know how much you know already about your relative's head injury; even if you have a lot of knowledge, it is likely that you will still have a few questions. We have written this section based on the questions that we are most often asked by people of your age. As you read this, if you have any further questions, write them down as they come to mind and ask an adult in the family, or someone else you trust, to help you find answers. The Internet has many useful websites about the brain and head injury and these are listed at the end.

What is a head injury?

A head injury is when the head and the brain get hurt or damaged. Head injury is also sometimes called a brain injury, a traumatic brain injury (TBI), or an acquired brain injury (ABI).

Who can get a head injury?

Anyone of any age can have a head injury.

Why does a head injury happen?

Most head injuries happen because of an accident. This could be a car accident (often called RTAs or road traffic accidents), a fall (perhaps off a ladder), or if the person is hit on the head by something (this can happen if the person is in a fight).

Even though there is usually an obvious cause of the injury, many children and young people blame themselves for it. They worry that they could somehow have caused it (this may seem like a strange idea but it is actually a very common worry). Some young people worry that the accident happened to 'pay them back' for things that they have done wrong (like arguing with their parents or getting into trouble at school). They also think that they might have been able to prevent the accident happening (by having done something differently on the day) or wish that they had been nicer to their relative before the injury.

It is important for you to know that your relative's injury did not happen because of anything you did and they would not want you to worry about this.

What happens when someone has a head injury?

Most people who have had a head injury will have to go to hospital where staff will work out how severe the injury is and decide on the best way to treat them.

Some people can go home after they have been checked out and will probably get better quite soon.

Some people, who have more serious injuries, will have to stay in hospital. They will usually need more tests (such as brain scans), be monitored to make sure they don't get worse, or have an operation on their brain. They might need to be transferred to ICU (intensive care) and then later move to another ward to recover. Waiting for them to be well enough to leave ICU can be very stressful; visiting them there can also be difficult as they might be unconscious (not awake or aware of what is happening around them), confused (and possibly not recognize you), or be attached to lots of machinery (e.g. to help them breathe).

This is a normal part of recovering from a head injury, but it can be upsetting and frightening to see your relative like this. Some young people don't want to visit the hospital—and this is OK. Find other ways of staying in touch with them instead, like sending cards.

People with head injuries might remain in hospital for many weeks or even months. They may have rehabilitation (treatments to help overcome some of the problems after the injury) in another hospital before they go home, or attend hospital clinics from home. Recovery is usually very lengthy.

Unfortunately, some people do not recover completely and can carry on having problems when they get home. This can be very stressful for everyone. A small number of people do not recover from their injury and, because they have so many problems, cannot go back home to live. Instead, they have to live in a place where they can be cared for by trained staff (such as a nursing home). It can be very sad when this happens, but usually everyone tries very hard to stay in touch and to visit.

Most people do not die because of a head injury, but a small number do. This might be due to the injury itself, or because of other problems that can develop afterwards, such as infections. Again, this is very hard for everyone in the family and they need a lot of support to cope with this.

What kinds of problems can people with head injuries have?

Because a head injury results in damage to the brain, people can have a wide range of problems:

- physical problems (e.g. cannot walk or use their arms)
- cognitive (thinking) problems (e.g. poor memory, problems concentrating, problems understanding what people say)
- emotional (feelings) problems (e.g. sadness, worry, depression, anger)
- behavioural (how we act) problems (e.g. being more aggressive, shouting, sitting still and doing nothing, doing or saying things quickly without thinking)
- relationship problems (e.g. arguing with relatives, ignoring others)

Sometimes these problems are so severe that the person seems very different to how they were before their injury. When these problems are very severe, the person cannot go back to work or be able to look after their family like they used to.

Understanding these problems can be very difficult—the injured person can look exactly the same as before the injury, but now they can act differently. Their behaviour can upset you, or make you angry or embarrassed, and you might not want your friends to see them like this. Sometimes, you might find things that they do funny, but they can get angry with you when you laugh at them.

Try to remember that they have changed because of the accident—not because they want to upset you, or because of anything you did. They still love you, even if it does not always seem like it.

The type of problems your relative will have depends on which parts of the brain have been injured. This is because different parts of the brain are responsible for or control different skills and abilities. However, the workings of the brain and what happens to it when it is injured are complex (and fascinating) topics. To learn more visit the www.washington.edu website. Enter 'Chudlar' into their home page search box and this will take you to 'Neurosciences for kids' where you can learn amazing facts about the brain.

Do head injury problems recover?

Yes—lots of problems after a head injury can improve. It can help if you can find ways of 'getting around' problems (like helping them use a calendar to remember things if they have a poor memory).

However, recovery from head injury can be lengthy, and even after many years people with head injuries can still have problems. If the injury was very severe, the person will probably have some problems for the rest of their lives. This can be upsetting as everyone wants them to return to 'normal'.

The problem is that it is very hard for doctors to work out who is going to get better and how long it will take. Usually we just have to wait and see what happens.

How does it feel to have a head injury?

It is difficult to answer this as we have not had a head injury. However, in our experience, people with head injures are usually upset and distressed about what has happened and worry about whether they will get better. They can be sad or angry about it all. If people have problems with their memory, they can feel very confused and might not be sure about what is going on.

However, some people are not as upset by having a head injury. This might be because they do not fully understand how serious their problems are or it could be because they have found helpful ways to cope with it.

Perhaps you could ask your relative about how they are feeling—or ask another adult to tell you more.

How does the rest of the family feel when a head injury happens?

Every family gets upset and worried when someone has a head injury. It can be a very difficult time for everyone, especially as no one is sure what is going to happen. Adults in the family may seem very sad or worried, and they might be away from the family home caring for your relative at the hospital. This can result in normal family activities stopping for a while. When the injured person comes home from hospital they might not be able to do the things they used to do, like drive the car or go to work, and so other people in the family might have to do these things instead. This can sometimes lead to tension and make people tired and upset. You might also be asked to do some extra jobs around the house to help out.

Sometimes the person with the head injury needs help to look after themselves, e.g. help having a bath or going to the toilet. If you are afraid that you will have to help them do these things, discuss this with an adult. It is important not to do things that make you feel uncomfortable.

There are many changes to get used to after a head injury and it can take time for things to feel OK again. It helps to tell someone when you are worried about anything.

How do young people feel when head injury happens in the family?

Not everyone feels the same about head injury. Some young people feel OK and can get on with their normal life. Others are much more worried and sad and find it hard to get on with things. They can find going to school very difficult and may not do as well with their work as they did before. This might be because worrying about their relative makes it hard to concentrate. Sometimes friends can ask difficult questions about the injured person or make hurtful comments about them, which are hard to handle.

Some young people find that they argue more with others in the family. They can have many worries—about the person who is ill, about the rest of the family, and about themselves. Being asked to do extra jobs around the house or to 'look after' the injured person can be very annoying, especially if this stops you from going out with your friends. There might also be less money coming into the house (if the injured person is not working) and so you might not be able to have the things you used to have. If friends notice, this it can be hard.

Feelings can get very mixed up. Some days you might feel sad; other days you might feel worried or guilty. Many young people feel angry that the accident happened and think that their life has been ruined, and it is common to want to get revenge on any other people involved in the accident. This can be a very strong and frightening feeling, but it is normal and many people feel like this for a while. The good thing is that these feelings don't last forever and will be easier if you tell someone about them.

Remember, there is no right or wrong way to feel about a head injury. Whatever you are feeling is OK.

What can help you feel better?

- Try to find out as much as you want to about how the brain works and what can go wrong when it is injured. Knowledge about head injury can make coping with it easier.
- Try to remember that none of this was your fault.
- Talk to an adult whom you like and trust about your worries, if you can. They will try to help you find ways to feel better about things. However,

young people often prefer to talk to friends or people outside the family about worries. If you can, tell your closest friends what is going on. Perhaps you could show them this book so that they can start to understand better. Is there a teacher at school you could talk to? You could also make an appointment to see your own family doctor who can talk about worries with you. If you do not want to speak to anyone face to face you could telephone Childline on 0800 1111. Your local branch of Headway, which is a charity that supports people with head injury and their families, might have family groups or groups for teenagers. They have a website (www.Headway.org.uk) that can tell you what is going on where you live. Many carers centres (see www.carers.org.uk to find out if there is one near you) also have groups for young people.

◆ It can help to write down any worries, feelings, or questions in a diary or journal. Later it can help to look back on the situation to see how things have changed.

◆ Try to remember that even though they have had an injury and may have changed, your relative still loves you.

Do you want to know more?

We hope that reading this has helped answer some of your questions. However, there will always be questions that we haven't been able to answer and we're sorry if we have missed yours out. It might help to speak to the adult who gave you this book. We also hope that reading this has not upset you. If it has made you feel worried, please talk to an adult straight away.

Ask your local library if they have any books about the brain. Also, here are some websites that you might want to look at:

◆ the website www.kidshealth.org has a great section called 'The brain is the boss' which teaches you how the brain works

◆ go to www.health.qld.gov.au which is a very good website for families (there is also a children's section called Brain Crew Kids Zone).

Glossary

Acceleration and deceleration injuries damage sustained when the brain is suddenly subjected to forces that throw it forwards and backwards inside the skull

Acute care hospital care provided soon after injury or illness

Acquired brain injury (ABI) any form of injury to the brain that is not congenital (i.e. not present at birth). It includes a range of conditions including stroke and head injury

ADL activities of daily living (such as bathing, dressing, eating)

Agnosia the loss of ability to recognize and identify previously well-known objects

Amnesia partial or complete loss of memory. The following terms are also used:

- Post traumatic amnesia (PTA) the time after head injury during which the person is confused and unable to take in new information
- Anterograde amnesia specific difficulties remembering events since the injury/illness
- Retrograde amnesia loss of memory for events prior to the injury/illness

Amygdala a cluster of nerve cells in the temporal lobes. The amygdala is part of the limbic system

Ankle–foot orthosis (AFO) a leg brace

Anterograde amnesia see amnesia

Anticonvulsants (or anti-epileptics) medication used to decrease the occurrence/recurrence of epileptic seizures

Aphasia (sometimes called dysphasia) aspeech and language disorder that can affect all aspects of language—understanding what is said to you, the ability to find words and sounds to speak, and the ability to read and write

Apraxia difficulty performing voluntary movements or actions (such as waving goodbye). Specific difficulties are experienced in thinking about and planning movements

Aspiration when food or fluids enter the lungs through the windpipe (this can lead to infection of the lungs or pneumonia)

Ataxia the arm or leg performs jerky and clumsy, uncoordinated movements. It is usually caused by damage to the cerebellum

Autonomic functions those bodily functions, such as heart rate and breathing, that are not under our voluntary control

Axons fibre-like parts of nerve cells that are used to send messages rapidly from one part of the brain to another

Basal ganglia cluster of nerve cells deep within the brain hemispheres which are involved in performing movements

Behaviour therapy a psychological approach to changing behaviour

Brain death the state when the brain stem permanently ceases functioning

Brainstem the part of the brain that is in charge of the body's most vital functions such as breathing, heart beat, wakefulness, and control of hormones

Capacity see mental capacity

Catheter a tube used to insert or withdraw fluids from the body (e.g. urinary catheter is used to withdraw urine from the bladder)

Central nervous system (CNS) the brain and the spinal cord make up the CNS

Cerebellum the part of the brain that plays a role in coordinating our movements

Cerebrospinal fluid (CSF) a watery fluid in and around the brain which provides it with some protection

Cerebrum The main part of the brain, which is made up of two hemispheres

Clonus rhythmic shaking of a limb caused by rapid contraction and relaxation of muscles

Closed head injury the most common head injury, in which the skull is not penetrated

Cognitive communication difficulties communication difficulties secondary to cognitive impairment (such as difficulties joining in a conversation because of reduced attention or slowed information processing speed)

Cognitive impairment problems with essential 'thinking abilities' such as problem-solving, memory, planning

Coma a state in which a person remains fully unconscious and unrousable

Compensatory techniques a range of strategies and aids that head-injured people are taught to use to reduce the impact of problems arising from the injury in everyday life (i.e. using a diary can compensate for having a poor memory)

Contractures stiffness in the soft tissues around joints, caused by shortening of muscle fibres and development of fibrous tissue in the surrounding soft tissues

Contrecoup injury in addition to the initial contusion at the site of impact, the brain is often also injured at the opposite side as it keeps wobbling back and forth

Contusion bruising of the brain. Cells of the brain are crushed and destroyed when they are thrown against the inside of the skull

Cortex the surface of the brain, which is involved in intellectual functioning. It contains billions of neurons

Cranium the skull

Crushing injury an injury that occurs when the head is compressed from two sides

CT scan computed tomography. A kind of X-ray examination which can show the brain and other parts of the body (also known as a CAT scan)

Deep vein thrombosis (DVT) blood clots that form in the veins, typically in the deep veins of the legs

Diffuse axonal injury widespread damage to the axons (the connections between nerve cells) in the brain

Disinhibition saying or doing things without thinking, being unable to control feelings

Disorientation being unable to know where you are, current date, etc.

Dysarthria a speech disorder caused by weakness of the muscles of speech or difficulty coordinating them. The speech sounds slurred and may be difficult to understand

EEG (electroencephalogram) the electrical activity of the brain is measured with electrodes on the surface of the skull. This is used to look for signs of epilepsy

Egocentric behaviour focusing on one's own needs and being unable to consider the needs of others

Emotional lability being unable to control emotions fully

Emotional numbness showing no emotions or a 'blunting' of emotional responses

Encephalitis inflammation of parts of the brain itself

Epilepsy recurring seizures (or fits/convulsions). Seizures occur when brain cells become over-excited and generate electrical impulses which spread erratically throughout the brain

Executive abilities a range of complex thinking processes such as planning, problem-solving, and control of behaviour and emotions

Extradural haematoma bleeding between brain surface and skull

Fibre-optic endoscopic evaluation of swallowing (FEES) a procedure in which a camera is passed up the nose and into the throat in order to observe muscle movement and residue when a patient swallows

Frontal lobes the part of the brain just behind the forehead. They are in charge of our higher-level thinking skills, initiating and planning our movements and actions. The left frontal lobe is necessary for speaking

Functional electrical stimulation (FES) a treatment method in physiotherapy which activates muscles with electric impulses

Gait pattern of walking

Gastrostomy feeding tube that is inserted into the stomach (through the wall of the abdomen) to provide nutrition to the patient

Glasgow Coma Scale (GCS) a simple method of measuring a person's level of consciousness

Grand mal epileptic seizure a person loses consciousness, falls to the ground, the body stiffens up, and both arms and legs go into violent shakes (also known as a tonic–clonic seizure)

Grey matter the cortex of the brain and some parts deep inside the brain with a high density of nerve cells

Haematoma bleeding caused by ruptures of blood vessels

Headway The UK's national head injury charity and support organization

Hemianopia a state in which patients cannot see what is on one side of their visual fields of both eyes—either on the right side in both eyes or the left side in both eyes

Hemineglect unawareness or lack of attention to one side (mostly the left) of space/the world around you. This can include lack of awareness of one side of the body

Hemiparesis weakness on one side of the body as a result of damage to the opposite side of the brain. The arm, the leg, and sometimes the face are weak on the same side

Hemiplegia paralysis on one side of the body

Hemispheres the two halves of the brain

Hydrocephalus collection of too much cerebrospinal fluid within and around the brain. This causes the pressure within the skull to increase

Hydrotherapy physiotherapy performed in a swimming pool

Hypothalamus part of the brain involved in regulating the body's 'internal environment' and keeping it in balance (e.g. it is involved in the control of blood pressure, body temperature, hormone release, hunger, and thirst)

ICP see intracranial pressure

ICU the intensive care treatment unit of a hospital which provides continual monitoring of patients who are in a serious condition after injury

Incontinence difficulty in controlling the bladder and bowels

Information processing speed (or thinking speed) the time taken to think through and process information

Intracerebral haematoma bleeding within the brain matter

Intracranial pressure (ICP) the pressure inside the skull, which can be increased in certain conditions such as oedema

Interdisciplinary professionals of different disciplines work together collaboratively to achieve shared patient goals. This is different from multi-disciplinary where professionals from different backgrounds work alongside each other (but not necessarily collaboratively) to achieve patient goals

Lightwriter a high-tech device that can help someone who is unable to speak to communicate

Limbic system parts of the brain that work together to produce what we experience as emotions or feelings

MRI (Magnetic Resonance Imaging) produces a picture of the brain using a strong magnetic field rather than X-rays. It provides a more detailed picture than a CT scan

Meningitis an inflammation of the membranes around the brain

Mental capacity Having the ability to make decisions (e.g. about financial affairs)

Mental Capacity Act 2005 new legislation in the UK to protect people who cannot make decisions for themselves. It provides clear guidelines for carers and professionals about who can take decisions in which situations

Minimally responsive state people who appear to have some, but little and fleeting, awareness of what is going on around them. They are not in a coma but neither are they fully alert

Motor functioning movement—includes both gross movements and fine motor skills

Nasogastric tube a plastic tube inserted through the nose into the stomach through which feeding is given

Neglect being unaware of one side of space (ignoring things on one side, or ignoring one side of the body). This is a form of attentional impairment

Neuro-rehabilitation rehabilitation within the context of neurological injury or illness (see rehabilitation)

Neuron a nerve cell—the brain is made up of billions of these

NICE guidelines recommendations for the prevention and treatment of ill health produced by the independent organization called the National Institute for Clinical Excellence (NICE)

Nystagmus jerky movements of the eyes usually due to damage to the brainstem

Occipital lobes situated at the back of the brain. They are involved in processing what we see

Oedema swelling of the brain by accumulation of too much water, usually caused by damage to the brain

Open head injury head injury caused when an object fractures and enters the skull, damaging the brain directly (also called a penetrating injury)

Paraparesis weakness in both legs

Parietal lobes located at the top of the brain. They are involved in feeling touch and pain, arithmetic, focusing our attention, and orientating ourselves

PEG (percutaneous endoscopic gastrostomy) a tube inserted surgically through the skin directly into the stomach. This allows a person to be fed over a long period

Penetrating head injury see open head injury

Perceptual functioning our ability to make sense of information coming in from our senses (i.e. what we see, hear, feel)

Permanent vegetative state a patient who stays in a vegetative (non-responsive) state over more than 12 months

Perseveration a pattern of thinking or behaving characterized by becoming fixed on, or returning repeatedly to, one topic or task and being unable to switch to an alternative

Persistent vegetative state a patient who stays in a vegetative (non-responsive) state for more than a month

Plasticity the ability of the brain to repair some of the damage that has happened in an injury

Pneumonia infection or inflammation of the lungs

Post-acute care care delivered once the individual is medically stable. This may occur in the hospital or in a rehabilitation setting

Post-concussion syndrome a group of symptoms including headache, dizziness, concentration problems, forgetfulness, and fatigue that commonly occur after mild head injury

Post-traumatic amnesia (PTA) the time after head injury during which the person is cofused and unable to take in new information (see amnesia)

Post-traumatic stress disorder (PTSD) an extreme form of anxiety disorder which can develop after a traumatic and life-threatening event. Symptoms of PTSD include emotional numbness, flashbacks to the event, nightmares, and a strong tendency to avoid reminders of the event

Pressure sores (or pressure ulcers) damage to the skin which occurs when an area of the body is exposed to pressure or friction for long periods of time

Prognosis the prospect of further recovery after illness or injury

Prospective memory your memory for things in the future (e.g. remembering to keep an appointment)

Reduced insight limited awareness of the changes that have happened to you after head injury

Rehabilitation an active dynamic process whereby an injured or ill person is helped to achieve their optimal level of functioning (see neuro-rehabilitation and vocational rehabilitation)

Reflex an involuntary and fast action (such as the knee jerk reaction) which does not involve the brain

Respite a temporary rest period from care responsibilities

Retrograde amnesia loss of memory for events prior to the accident/injury (see amnesia)

Rotation injury injuries that occur when the brain turns inside the head suddenly and quickly

Sedation giving someone medication to put them to sleep or calm them down

Seizures fits or convulsions (see epilepsy)

Spasm short-lasting stiffening or jumping of a limb

Spasticity stiffness of an arm or leg (also called increased muscle tone)

Stroke occurs when the blood supply to the brain is disrupted in some way (e.g. due to a blocked blood vessel) leading to brain cell damage and death

Subdural haematoma bleeding between the brain surface and the skull

Suprapubic catheter a plastic tube that is inserted surgically through the abdominal wall into the bladder

Temporal lobes located at the sides of the brain. They are involved in hearing, understanding language, and memory

Tetraparesis weakness in all four limbs (also called quadriparesis)

Tinnitus a sensation of ringing or buzzing in the head which is not related to noise outside

Total communication a way of communicating involving more than just speech. It involves encouraging all means of communication, including gesture, facial expression, written words, and drawings

Tracheostomy an artificial opening made in the windpipe (through surgery) to allow breathing

Traumatic brain injury (TBI) sudden-onset brain injury caused by trauma such as falling, car accident, or assault

Tremor rhythmic shaking of a limb

Vegetative state the patient has no apparent awareness of what is happening to them, but the body still keeps the heart beating and often the breathing going. A kind of sleep–wake cycle develops

Ventilation if a person cannot breathe for themselves, a machine (ventilator) will do it for them by regularly pumping air into their lungs

Vocational rehabilitation rehabilitation focused on helping people to resume work following illness or injury (see rehabilitation)

Ventricles spaces within the brain that are filled with fluid (see cerebrospinal fluid)

Verbal dyspraxia difficulty in programming and sequencing the movements of speech muscles to make speech sounds and sequence them in words

Vestibular system helps to keep equilibrium or balance

Videofluoroscopy examination of swallowing using X-rays

Vital signs blood pressure, heart beat, breathing sounds of the lung, and temperature

White matter areas of the brain that are made up of nerve cell fibres connecting other brain areas

Young carer refers to children and young people under the age of 18 who are providing significant and regular amounts of care

Index